DISSOLVING THE ENIGMA

of

DIVINE HEALING

By

Dr. Rev. Christopher Macklin

Published By: Christopher Macklin Ministries Inc.

To contact Christopher Macklin:

Telephone: (1) 417-334-6200

Email: info@christophermacklinministries.com

Web Address: www.christophermacklinministries.com

Other Products by Christopher Macklin Ministries include:
See Web Site for details

Printed in the United States of America

First Edition, First Printing 2014

ISBN

Cover Design By: Ginelle Macklin (Known as "The Nelly")

Edited By: Elaine J. Keller

Concepts presented in this book derive from Divine Love, Knowledge and Absolute Faith. They are not to be understood as directions, recommendations or prescriptions of any kind. Nor does the author or publisher make any claim to do more than provide information and report the information.

Acknowledgements

I am so excited that the book is now finally published. I would like to thank "The Nellie" (my wife) for all the support she has given me in the ministry and helping me with ideas on the book.

I would also like to thank Elaine J. Keller for her typing of my dictation and her excellent editing skills, as well as all of her amazing ideas.

I would like to thank Vaishali & Elliot for their amazing support of our ministry and with the forward of this book.

I would also like to thank Sarah for her time with proofreading (and input) regarding this book.

I would like to thank all of our clients for their continued support of us and the ministry. Thank you for allowing us to be a part of your healing process.

I would like to thank God and The Universe for working with me on a daily basis to facilitate the healings.

Sending out our Unconditional Love in the utmost capacity to our family, friends & clients for all that they are in our lives!

Table of Contents

Chapter 4: Causes of Illness and How to Heal Them

Chapter 5: The Divine Healing Modalities

Chapter 6: Illnesses A to Z

Alzheimer's

Aorta Valve, Arteries, Calcification, Hardening of the Arteries (also see Heart)

Arthritis, Bone Spurs

Autism

Blood Disorders

Brain Aneurisms, Strokes

Breast Cancer

Cancer, all forms, including Brain, Liver and all forms of Lymphoma

Candida, Thrush

Diabetes, Hypoglycemia

Emotional Conditions, including Bipolar, Manic depression, Personality Disorders

Eye Issues, including Cataracts, Macular Degeneration, Blindness, Myopia and TON

Fibromyalgia

Gall Bladder

Genetic "defects" causing Cystic Fibrosis, Huntington's, Parkinson's, Muscular Dystrophy, Rheumatoid Arthritis, Creutzfeldt-Jakob Disease, Downs syndrome, Epilepsy, Hodgkin's Disease, and Spinal Bifida

GI, Wheat Intolerance, Food Intolerance, Colon, Stomach, Intestinal Issues, IBS, Crohns, Reflux, Celiac

Hearing Loss c

Bacterial and Viral Infections, including Meningitis, Herpes, Epstein Barr, Mononucleosis

Heart Issues, MVP, Mitochondrial Disease, Pulmonary Edema

Hormonal Disorders (male and female), Menopause, PMS, Post Partum Depression

Interdimensional Implants

Kidney and Adrenal Issues

Leukemia, Liver Disorders, Lupus, Gout, Cirrhosis

Loss of Spirituality, Low Spiritual Awareness

Lung Defects, Chronic Bronchitis, Emphysema, Tuberculosis

Lyme Disease, the stealth pathogen Borrelia, AIDS /HIV

Morgellons Syndrome

Neuropathy, Nerve Ending Damage

Obesity & Weight Issues

Operation Problems, Tattoos, Surgery, Piercings

Osteoporosis

Phantom Pain

Conclusion

Testimonials

Prayers

Foreword

"Macklin Magic"

Face to face, Christopher Macklin is an ordinary, actually quite disarming man. Underneath that suave and demure exterior resides a man of extraordinary spiritual and physical healing abilities. Describing them would be like trying to shove the entire Solar system through a rabbit hole. So, those of us in the "biz" just refer to them as "Macklin Magic".

Chris would be the first person to admit that healing is the direct result of a person's relationship with their own Divine Nature; and that dis-ease is caused by the lack of a quality relationship in a person's life, with that Divine Nature. We could add incense, burning candles, sitar music and all wear white linen robes… but that's not what Chris is about. He shakes things up; he laughs and jokes during sessions. He is the person you'd most want to go out and have a drink with. He doesn't hold back. He not only understands life; he lives what he teaches. Who says spirituality has to be dull and slow moving? I suggest you fasten your seat belts, because even his prayers take a different perspective: "… I command you, God…" Hey! Why not? If I'd have said that, my parents would have sent me to military school. Oh! Wait! They did. Too bad I didn't know Christopher then.

As a spiritual teacher I have spent my entire adult life sharing one of the single most important Spiritual Laws: ***You are what you love and you love whatever you give your attention to***. This Law is important, but what is just as important is how to incorporate this Law into your daily life, in order to take your power back - spiritually, physically, mentally, emotionally and financially. Simple, right?

When you give your attention to limited things, you get limited results. It's the direct and immediate consequence of your love for what is limited. Christopher's work allows you to see how you have reacted to these self-imposed constrictions and then rise above them. "Macklin Magic" has been described as gently and lovingly realigning your Soul's direction with all that is good and true. But from my personal experience it's more like, "Hey Boys, we're moving in and taking control. The party's over. Grab you sh*t and hit the road." Obviously you get what you need when you need it. After all it's Macklin Magic, which means it is exactly right for the needs of each and every individual.

The "Macklin Magic" is what happens when you choose to welcome this good resident of Heaven and his sharing into your field of attention. The "Magic" support, wisdom and healing can come in the form of a one-to-one session with Christopher, reading this book, taking one of his classes or workshops, or listening to his radio interviews. Any way you get it, it's "Macklin Magic."

I encourage you to decide for yourself. If you've gotten this far in the Foreword, you might as well just go ahead and buy the book. Clearly you were meant to. The "Macklin Magic" is in your hands now! You can change your world. We have!

~ Vaishāli & Elliot Malach, author, and publishers of *You Are You What You Love*® book and radio series and *Wisdom Rising* & *Wisdom Rising II*

Preface

Who is Christopher Macklin and how did he come to Divine Healing?

In an English town somewhere near the Welsh Border, a boy sleeps.

Frightening creatures penetrate his dreams. Reptilian scales, red eyes, and malicious souls...the creatures inch closer, trying to grip him with their pointed talons. His cries freeze in his throat until his screams eventually break free and bring his mother to his side.

"Not again, Chris?" his mother exclaims when she reaches him. "Try to relax," she says, doing her best to soothe him, adding, "It's only your imagination."

"You'd best ring the doctor," Chris's father suggests as he enters the room. "These episodes," he says, referring to Chris' nighttime visitations, "are becoming altogether too frequent."

Young Chris knows the doctor won't help him. He knows no one can understand what is going on. He knows only one thing that will help, and for that he must become strong and very focused.

The household Christopher Macklin was born into was not a particularly religious one. Talk of spiritual matters centered on a distant heaven and hell much the same as it did in other homes in this middle class neighborhood. Chris, his brother, and parents, attended church on Sundays where the pastor extolled about God's magnanimity, and instructed followers on how to repent for their sins. These things made little impression on Chris, whose thoughts from an early age centered on weightier matters, matters like what made things evil, what made things good, and if there was a heaven and hell, weren't people already in them here on earth?

Soon enough, young Chris came to recognize the nighttime visitations for what they were: malicious beings trying to stop him from doing something important and good. He knew this because the "downloads" had begun. Hazy morning memories revealed lessons learned the previous nights, instructional sessions that infused him with knowledge of things he'd never previously heard of. He knew something out of the ordinary was happening when he awoke feeling like he'd run a marathon. As opposed to the evil episodes with the scaly creatures, these learning experiences were, despite their exhausting nature, filled with light. He knew he was attending a type of school and that he was being educated for a specific purpose, a purpose that had to do with healing.

"Everyone has their talent," the adult Reverend Macklin says. Whether it's painting, writing, expressing through music, curing illness, educating, or in some way creating and bettering humanity, each individual has a true gift and soulful purpose. His personal mission, Christopher came to realize, was to heal and educate humanity. A darkness was enshrouding the world, one that was not actively being addressed by any known religion or healing method. This darkness was pervading all things and was meant to prevent humanity from evolving. As the current earth cycle approached its close, it signaled the birth of a spiritually renewed, loving, and God-realized humanity, causing those on the dark side to increase efforts to keep humanity under its control. People needed to learn how to rise in their own divinity and divest themselves of emotional infirmities, mental distractions and physical illnesses that ailed them, and to call upon the highest God of the Universe powers of Unconditional Love, in order to keep this darkness in check. This is what was needed for humanity to triumph.

Over the years Christopher Macklin's downloads expanded. He learned that he is a Melchizedek spliced being here as one of the earth's spiritual guardians. The Melchizedeks are part of the order of Magi kings who recognized the arrival of Christ, and whose efforts to help humanity have spanned epochs. This organization helps produce profound healing through manifestation and absolute faith in the Universal Creator. Christopher came to realize that people misunderstand absolute faith. You can manifest death by fear, or you can manifest a positive reality through absolute faith. Where other methods fail is in overlooking the essential nature of complete, blind, unwavering faith.

As far as being "spliced," Macklin explains that his soul split at birth and entered two bodies at once. If this and other ideas discussed here seem farfetched, this book will help clarify things. In any case it is up to you, as reader, to accept or reject information according to your own inner compass. There is no right or wrong as long as you accept that which you feel is correct, and not reject new thoughts simply because someone else calls them "silly," "impossible," or anything less than Godly.

Chris Macklin has made an effort not to read books or hear others talk about subjects related to who he is and what he does so as to not affect the information he receives. His understanding is that Melchizedek beings are from the ultimate dimension and sit with the God of the Universe. The reptilian creatures that once invaded his nights and who are trying to prevent humanity from evolving are especially vicious in going after those who are spiritually awake and who firmly know what they are here to do. For this reason, he and others trying to work in the light become ready targets. Protection must be increased not only for those in need of healing, but for the healers as well.

As for myself, I first met Reverend Christopher Macklin in the fall of 2012. I'd been raised in a holistic and spiritual family, so it wasn't out of the norm for my mother to suggest I utilize the services of a psychic healer she'd heard about. I had been experiencing severe lower back pain for several years at that juncture, and had exhausted nearly every avenue of non-traditional healing I could find. I was at the point of attempting to live with the pain, which isn't something I was happy about. Enter Chris Macklin. He explained where the blockage was coming from, why it was there, and how to get rid of it. I quizzed him mercilessly, for as a writer and hard-core researcher I refuse to let any subject go until understanding it to my satisfaction. My work had taken me to some pretty far-out places by this time, and because of my family, my experience with holistic healing and psychic healers was vast. What Christopher explained with regard to what he was doing and why, resonated profoundly within me. I believed then, and still do, that very few people if any, are addressing such imperative things as he is, and certainly not in such a direct, effective, and courageous approach.

As far as my spinal issues, the healing would likely need four sessions, Chris explained, spaced over a period of a couple of months. He said that I would have to pray every two hours while the healing was in progress, without fail. When I neglected to rigorously uphold this protocol, the pain quickly resurfaced. I didn't make that mistake again.

After one session what had been chronic, debilitating pain lessened by a good 30% before reverting to what it had been beforehand, returning, I suspect, because of my erratic prayers. After two sessions the pain was down 50%. After three it was nearly gone. After four sessions it was gone completely, never to return. That is, I won't let it return, now that I know how to keep it at bay.

As my relationship with Christopher continued in the form of obtaining help for loved ones, I naturally quizzed him on every possible occasion. When he mentioned he had been trying to write a book but due to time constraints hadn't thus far accomplished it, I examined my own schedule and questioned my sanity in jumping into the fray. It is a book that has to be written, as you will soon see, for his understanding of the world we find ourselves in now, and his approach to dealing with the illnesses that result, is unlike anything you will hear or read about elsewhere.

I consider it a privilege and great blessing that Chris has allowed me to share in the writing process with him. I wish freedom and good health to each one of you.

In Love & Light,
Elaine J. Keller

~ Elaine J. Keller, author of *Light Your Fire, The Ayurveda Diet for Weight Loss, Tale of Running Bear, Mother's Guide to the New World Order Series, and more.*

INTRODUCTION

In the Author's Words

Absolute faith is the true and powerful secret that governs our lives. When you have absolute faith nothing can touch you. This is a knowing inside, with no fear and complete confidence in God, that nothing can or will harm you. Any slight fear can prevent absolute faith, while it is strengthened by direct connection with God, talking directly to Him, meditating, praying, and asking for His protection.

Faith, as you may well know, will overcome the seemingly worst of situations. During my lifetime journey I spent twenty years in the corporate world. Though I reaped great material benefit, I didn't fit in well there and found it very difficult to work in an environment where manipulation and negativity were normal occurrences. I never understood this fully until losing my family, my home, and all life's "comforts" when going bankrupt. These jarring events brought me to a point of desperation whereupon I called upon God to prove himself.

If you are in the third dimensional world making a salary, you are most likely not expanding your gifts. The God realm lets you be, for you must determine your own journey. You may think you are on the right path but in truth you are led by ego. This is what happened to me. I needed to go back and meditate my ego away, and this I did, day and night for weeks, months, and years. The journey we think we are on isn't necessarily the path God wants us to follow. For those concerned about sitting in the lotus position while trying to still your restless mind, rest assured that meditation takes many forms. Walking, painting, being silent, or doing whatever relaxes you and causes your thoughts to unfold will allow an inner knowing of things to come through.

Once you understand your gifts and begin your journey on the God path, blessings come to you every day. Not just monetarily, but through the blessing of giving your talents to other people, healing, changing them for the better, and uplifting them. Money is energy. You can use money for good or for bad; it is your choice. Used for good it can bless people's lives. Yet it's important to discern whether people want or will allow change in their lives. When we bless people, I always say, "allow the blessing to flow down the line." It's important to give from your heart and to never have any expectations in return.

Sometime after leaving the corporate world, I began healing others. I manifested sponsors and was able to travel the world teaching and healing. My journey took me to India, Gambia, Ghana, Belize, and America. People responded very well. They were being healed, and as they gained understanding, they were able to experience joy in living. Every morning now, I awaken feeling blessed and excited to be alive with the feeling of universal love and protection, thanks to being able to use my gifts.

When we come here, to the 3D world, it's with the purpose of learning absolute faith and Christ Consciousness. The true definition of Christ Consciousness is living in the space of Absolute Faith, with no fear, and with Unconditional Love for every living being on this planet. People talk casually about *Unconditional Love*, but not everyone takes the time to understand what being in this space really entails. Unconditional Love means to truly put yourself in another person's shoes and send him or her positive, loving energy from your heart without judgment, whether he is a beggar, a family member or a terrorist.

Letting Go in the Now

When you're in need of healing, and this includes almost everyone, it's important to come before God and release any karma you've accrued during this lifetime. You don't have to go to a priest; you have to ask God for forgiveness from your heart for whatever has gone on down here. Clearing karma means forgiving yourself for the wrongdoing and asking God for forgiveness, and sending Unconditional Love to the individuals who may have been harmed. We only have Unconditional Love here; there is nothing else. All other emotions are brought about by manipulations that send you on the wrong path.

Unreleased karma creates illness. Sometimes we have illness because

God wants us back on his side. If you are not learning down here, then God will take you back. If you learn and release the illness then you can change your body's vibration to a high vibrational state. No disease can live in a high vibration body. Low vibration can be brought about by the toxicity of what's going on in this planet. You need to release and remove the toxins before being able to reach that high vibrational state. Much, if not all of the illness we experience on this planet comes from manipulation. The things that cause disease are toxins, emotions, and transmission frequencies. These affect the body as well as our vibrational state. Two are caused by manipulation, and one is affected by manipulation. Some are self-induced. All of this will be gone over in the following sections.

As I said, God can take us back early because we're not learning down here. It's vital to release that karma and receive God's forgiveness. It's important to live in the now, and not be put off your path of self-discovery or of using your gifts. Doing this takes complete *letting go.* Take a look at what's in the here and now and understand that you are blessed. Take a step back and let God do the work—for He will. Even the negative things that occur in your life create blessings, and knowingly accepting these blessings while understanding their purpose is part of Absolute Faith.

Living in the now is important because what you do right now is everything. We have free will. You can live in hell on earth, or heaven on earth. Hell is right here, right now. Hell is a world of fear, misery, gossip, illness, making money for its own sake, and despair. Why are so many people who work for others miserable? Because their job is not serving their purpose or utilizing their true gifts. If you release all your fear and live in Absolute Faith, everything will come to you.

When you've done all your work on this planet then it's time to move on, or, if you're failing to learn, the Creator Gods will take you back and put you back here to learn again.

Third dimensional belief often takes the form of dogmatic religion, and puts us in a space of judgment and containment. It's important to let go of all the things you've been taught to think and look at the ascended master's teachings with an open mind. Jesus taught this, as did Buddha, Hay Baba, Babaji, Toth, and all ascended masters.

I realized I was gifted by the age of four. I could see inter-dimensional spirits. I was visited by anunnaki and the greys. During the reptilian visits I could feel their low vibrational darkness. When they visited I didn't understand what they were, but they had a profound effect on me. My parents didn't understand why I had so many bad dreams. They said "don't worry, it's just a bad dream, go back to sleep." They didn't realize I was being visited by the dark entities.

Understanding is a kind of download. When you go to sleep, you get a lot of information. There's no time in the other dimensions. You could be there for twenty years in one night. When you wake up you might feel exhausted. That's because you've been educated. A lot of times you don't know you've been educated, you just feel it. It's important to go with gut feelings and have faith in that knowing.

I soon learned what my visitors were and why they were here, and also how to block them. I was given divine prayers to remove them. They were visiting me to try and shut me down, so I wouldn't achieve the teachings and healings I was put here to do.

These divine prayers were the beginning of what I was to receive, and part of what I share with you here. The other is spiritual understanding and a way to cure illness. If your vibration is not high enough it's dangerous to practice these techniques. Once your vibration drops from stress, for instance, it lowers your defenses and negative energy can come in. Prayers and direction are given on how to combat this.

When I received downloads I didn't allow negativity inside. Although I was always gifted my true knowledge came when I went bankrupt in England. I was allowed to meditate for three years, which is how I came to understand who and what I've been for the last four thousand years, and what I've done that has brought me to the now with expanded gifts and teachings. I am a spiritual teacher and healer, spliced as a Melchizedek being.

In this lifetime I am supposed to help people expand their minds about dogma and religions and help them shift to a new conscious Godlike state which will change the very fabric of their existence to one of Unconditional Love and high vibration. There's an old saying that harkens back to the Knights Templar and King Arthur, "The truth will set you free." There are many people on the planet who are teachers, but who are being manipulated. I am able to bypass the manipulation because of my complete understanding. Unless you clear the channels properly, your intent will be influenced by negativity. I have demonstrated the technique for doing this all over the world.

In the past several years my most profound experience was in Belize, meditating upon the Mayan temples. All Mayan temples are built on ley lines so they possess a very strong energy which allows your vibration to heighten and your consciousness to expand. They are still effective despite tampering. Many things have been affected by manipulation. They showed me visions of my past lives then, which were very powerful.

What You will Find in This Book

You have to live by your gut feeling. That's the most powerful tool you have. If your inner feeling is that this book is correct, then it's for you. If it's not correct then that's okay. That's your reality.

This world we live in is indeed very much like the Matrix movie. We exist in a surreal ecosphere of vibration that allows you to change anything around you, as long as you have absolute belief. *The Secret* explains about belief, but it doesn't take manipulation and blockages into consideration. We will explain this further here as well as in upcoming books, and provide a technique for countering these blockages. This technique is called *Rapid Divine Magi Manifestation*. It protects us from manipulation and allows us to manifest from the God realm with the use of sacred geometry and angelic writing. The high vibration of sacred geometry blocks out negativity completely. Angelic writing speeds the request onward to God in the highest realm.

Everything depends on vibration in this surreal world. Your body can vibrate high or low, like water. There is a correlation between the vibration of water, crystal, and gold, and this is why gold is very good for your body. Yet gold powder can produce the reverse effect. If you've got entity blockages and take gold the entity gets worse. Gold is good only when you've cleared. Clearing is an essential part of the process, and is explained further in these pages.

We are going to teach you how to be in the God Space and the techniques to use for energy healing. Most people's perception of energy healing is Reiki, a universal life force energy dealing with the 3rd dimension. The problem with this is that the 3D vibration is blocked and not as effective as it once was. In this third dimensional world the vibration is dropping and therefore the universal life force is dropping also. To combat this we now need to tap into inter-dimensional energies, which are far more stronger. This energy is sought through inter-dimensional portals. It is very important to get permission to access this energy first. This will be explained further in the book.

The energies, what they are, and much more will be described in the following pages.

It is my sincere hope that you find the information presented here informative, uplifting, and healing. At the very least, I hope that it in some manner it improves your lives, and helps you fulfill the purpose you were born to do. Each of us has important gifts. Understanding which dimension you came from and tapping into that dimension for help, will help get you into a high vibrational state with Absolute Faith, Inner Peace And Unconditional Love. This is my wish.

With Unconditional Love and Blessings,
Dr. Rev. Christopher Macklin

CHAPTER 1

The Dimensions

Earth as we experience it exists in the third dimension. This 3D world is a learning center, along with the first, second, and fourth dimensions. Our lessons and experiences here are meant to advance our spirituality with the assistance of free will, and this is what seems to be at the heart of the issue—the issue being, that when people turn to greed or ego-centered consumption they fail to love others as much as themselves. The world has gotten into a mess because of lack of Unconditional Love and compassion along with an increased level of fear. Fear should have no place in our beings. It is manufactured by those in control to keep us in a state of tyranny.

Governmental agents and the large families who control 99.99% of the wealth of this planet have engineered a world they can control through illness, debt, and most of all, fear. One of the largest families controls nine-hundred thousand trillion dollars. With this sort of wealth you can buy the media, presidents, kings and queens, and every world ruler. Greed and selfishness comes in when we allow these families to control virtually everything about us, a phenomenon we will go into in greater depth further on.

In the first four dimensions you can live in heaven or hell depending upon what your choice is. Living in heaven is letting go completely. This means not worrying about money but going forward on the God Path with all of your gifts. These gifts may entail healing, instructing, painting, music, or expressing creativity of any sort. Creativity increases God's vibrational flow. Stimulating artwork imbues people with joy and is healing. A gifted teacher infuses students with passion, soaring spirit, and understanding. Even some in the corporate world might be using their gifts in a creative way. A chef heals with dishes and herbs, eliciting a wow factor that increases people's vibrations. If you are unhappy in your present occupation you are likely not using your gifts and knowledge fully.

The fifth dimension is where the Creator Gods come from. The Creator Gods consist of Pleiadians, Arcturians, Andromedans, and Sumerians and exist in Orion's Belt. They are guided by a galactic federation consisting of many types of light beings, and which is headed up by the Melchizedek order from the other dimensions, with Jesus, the Christ Soul, being the ultimate Melchizedek Being. There are infinite dimensions and He takes many forms within many different dimensions at one time.

The Creator Gods came down here to build the pyramids as telephone devices so we could meditate and connect to them. These were shut down by the dark side, and their interface mechanisms were removed. This device is the *merkaba*, a crystal energy accelerator which was located atop the pyramids and which is the true ark of the covenant. The Creator Gods wanted to create a race of unconditionally loving beings that had been given the gift of free will in order to see what they would do. They didn't anticipate the level of manipulation the malevolent inter-dimensional beings would use to interfere on our path of Unconditional Love. The Creator Gods have empowered us to overcome this, but our emotions leave us susceptible to manipulation. The Creator Gods work with us as long as we are on the right path, but when we persist on the wrong path they must let us find the way for ourselves. Federation rules stipulate that every individual must create his own journey.

People often wonder why God isn't coming down and helping us. The answer is that God *is* helping. If you ask, you will receive. You have to ask with authority. There are a number of starseeds being born down here now with souls from the Creator Gods. These beings of the light are born to help at this time because we are heading for a big change. When these souls are born they are manipulated on a daily basis. Starseeds must take extra effort to protect themselves. There is more on starseeds later in the book.

The Creator Gods spliced the human race in order to put us down here, splitting off over 50 genes from various Creator Gods and souls of light and love in order to create the ultimate being. When you leave here after your lifetime, your soul goes back to the Creator Gods, who effectively allow you to re-experience the lifetime and emotions of what your actions created, both good and bad. In other words, when you pass on, you will experience the impact you've had on others, and learn how well you did with the journey during the last lifetime.

People ask about the Akashic Records, which are located in the 5th dimension. These soul maps hold the patterns of many lifetimes and cannot be touched. However, if you tap into them the answer can be manipulated by entities that alter the information. It's very important to clear the channel before you ask any and all questions. Precede questions with, "In the name of God," as fallen angels and dark souls don't like the name of God and will detach themselves, at least temporarily. You have a maximum of thirty seconds to get the right answer before they come back.

If you look at your life, every day is a crossroads. We have a choice of going one way or another. Choosing the God path is usually not the easiest, but it's the correct one.

Once you've experienced this lifetime and return to the 5th dimension you can ask to come back down here and focus on the part of the journey that you didn't understand or get right. There is no time in the 5th dimension. When you are born there is no karma. You come back here by choice because you want to improve the parts of the lifetime that need rebalancing through new experience and new choices. You come here each time with a clean slate, ready to experience a new lifetime and learn the things you didn't understand before. We are born here to experience a new journey. God is Unconditional Love, and forgives you before you do anything wrong. Thus the idea of "bad karma," or "repaying debts," is incorrect.

There is a subtle difference between karma and choice. Karma is less important than the journey and the experience of free will and choice. Balancing karma by reliving the journey to experience those parts of the lifetimes you didn't get correct isn't mandatory, but most people elect to come back and expand their spiritual growth. The Creator Gods allow you to come back again until you do things correctly and move into a Christ Conscious state. In this respect, karma exists.

When you are with unconditional loving beings in the 5th dimension they point things out to you. They want you to experience growth and to get to an unconditionally loving, Christ state where you have absolute faith. Suicide happens when people who can't maintain the journey are ordered back. If you don't see the whole lifetime through, you return right away. The things you got wrong can be focused on next time around. If you didn't achieve Absolute Faith you will have to go back because you are on a journey to expand your consciousness. Ascension is attaining Christ Consciousness and transferring to the 5th dimension.

The way to ascend is to adopt Unconditional Love and Complete Faith.

The higher dimensions house many light beings. Some are governed by free will and others are light dimensions, while Melchizedek beings sit in the ultimate dimension. Their responsibility is policing the universe in all of its dimensions to help where they can, to guide people and improve their spiritual growth. There's five of these beings on this planet now, working within multiple dimensions, striving for the ultimate good of mankind.

In the ultimate, infinite, dimension is the highest God of the Universe, the Creator of All That Is, and He is governed by Unconditional Love. This is the God that many people believe in and know by different names.

It's important when discovering your gifts to uncover which dimension you're from. You will need to get permission to connect to the Creator Gods of your dimension. Ask these Gods, who are extensions of God of the Universe, and they will help you. If you go poking in the wrong dimension nothing will happen because you haven't gotten permission to be there. That's why meditation and connecting to your higher self when discovering your gifts is important. There are many lifetimes going on in different dimensions at one time. You can be on many planets in many dimensions at once, but each lifetime is connected to your higher self. Your higher self exists in one dimension. This is the dimension you need to connect with.

While karma doesn't transfer from past lifetimes we are getting *esoteric transference* because the veil is thinning between the 3rd and 5th dimensions. The negative entities that are manipulating us are located in the first, second and most significantly, in the fourth dimension. The interference by entities is explained further on in the book. For now, understand that we are ascending directly to the fifth dimension in a two-dimensional shift.

Esoteric transference is when things that are embossed on your soul pass through lifetimes, because the veil is so thin. This is not karma, but accidental transference. Although karma is reset from one lifetime to the next, memories and impressions from past lives pass through by way of this transference, through your soul and cellular memory. Memory embossed on the cell that is still prominent must be removed in order to alleviate blockages. This is done through past life clearing and prayer. Always say these prayers three times as the most sacred numbers are 3 and 9. Every time you say the prayer you should feel lightness come over your body. If you don't feel this shift after the third time, say the prayer nine times.

Prayer to Release Cellular Memory or Esoteric Transference from Past Lives

I am of God

I ground myself to the earth

I come before you now, God,

for forgiveness for anything I have done

in any past life to infinitum

through all space/time continuum in every dimension

that has been brought back into this lifetime

and is affecting me now

I release it all to You, God,
with Unconditional Love.

I thank You, God,

and send You my Unconditional Love

So Be It
Amen

Cellular memory needs to be cleared because it affects your body's vibration. When we are born, every woman on this planet has an esoteric crystal structure around her womb that is not visible but which is extremely important to the birthing process. When the sperm hits the egg, the soul is transferred through this esoteric structure via the fifth dimension, and bonds with the egg and sperm. Many women are struggling with becoming pregnant because an attachment in the abdomen is damaging the esoteric structure and preventing the new soul from passing through. We'll share in the healing chapters how to correct this. When sperm hits the egg it has 48 hours to attach the soul. If the soul fails to attach, the fertilized egg will abort because it is not a complete being, in other words, a being without a soul. The soul that's assigned to that sperm and egg will come back to someone else. If someone has an abortion the soul will be born again. Miscarriage occurs when the soul doesn't properly bond with the egg. It's a spiritual process. Sometimes there is a dark entity in the womb creating the miscarriage causing the vibration of the baby to drop.

It is important that we learn Absolute Faith during this lifetime. How would you feel if a gunman came into your room, pointed the gun, and began squeezing the trigger? Ninety-nine percent of us would be overcome by fear, which is the wrong response. Absolute Faith prevents anything negative from touching you. You are protected full stop. With absolutely no doubt you know that the universe will create a new reality where you will not die from that gunshot. The gun will become jammed or the gunman will have a heart attack. *Something* will occur to prevent the worst from happening.

In the bible one of the disciples drank poison and remained alive because he had *Absolute Faith*. I tested God myself, during a low point following my bankruptcy. I wanted to explore my faith in God and God's faith in me. After all, it's a joint partnership. The outcome of that test is that I am still here, but I remember the episode vividly. It's not something I recommend, and I beg you not to try it yourself. Suffice to say that I subjected my body to a toxic substance that should have killed me several times over. I became physically sick. I couldn't get enough water. I felt like I'd demolished my liver. I was alone in a hotel room, which suddenly filled with angels. One of the angelic beings said to me, "You're going nowhere." I recognized him as Archangel Michael. God had visited me and was showing me

Unconditional Love.

I was led to this path with my eyes wide open to cement my relationship with God. This was a confirmation of my Absolute Faith. I had told God that if he wanted me to do His work, then I wanted to see a demonstration. Likewise I would take poison to show my Absolute Faith that God would keep me here. Without God's intervention, I wouldn't be here. Anyone who hasn't got 100% Absolute Faith will pass on. It's like passing your hand through a solid wall: believe, and your hand will pass through unscathed; panic, and your molecular shape will change causing your hand to become trapped inside the wall. Gifts like this are only given to people who are ready to receive with Absolute Faith, the highest vibration, and with Unconditional Love. Your God realm won't allow you to do things you are not ready for. Like I said, don't try this at home.

While the main dimensions we're involved in are one through five, there are many different types of beings and planets within these dimensions. I feel it's important to cover the ones that primarily affect us.

The 1st and 2nd Dimensions

In the first dimension, there are lots of insect-type creatures. They look like scarab beetles and jellyfish forms in their own dimension, but become energy fields once they enter our reality. They can get into the body and affect our meridian flow. These parasites are only slightly dark yet cause harmful blockages. People wonder why they get arthritis on one side of their body and not the other. This is because blockages stop the flow on one side or the other, causing bones to crystallize. Doctors seem to think arthritis comes with old age. Don't believe it. These forms which take shape in our dimension as energy fields are at fault.

The second dimension gives rise to snake beings. Often they get in the body, sit on a shoulder, or in a breast or hip, especially in those of the ladies. It's difficult to tell if they're there. When we send in high vibrational energy there's a tightening reflex.

Removal of these entities must be of high vibration or they will come back. To keep them away your body must be in a high-vibrational state. This is the crux of the matter when dealing with all forms of low vibrational entities. We'll cover how to accomplish this later.

Snakes and other beings cannot get into a high vibrational body. If you have emotional issues of any sort, or if your emotions are precarious, the entity can get in and affect your body. In their dimension these entities manifest as actual bodies, while in this dimension they are low vibrational energy fields. If you have acquired one of these low-vibe entities, in the breast, for instance, it will block the whole breast allowing a fungal infection to set in, and in which cancer may result. We will explain the healing process for this later.

The 4th Dimension

Fourth dimensional beings who primarily affect us are zeta greys, anunnaki reptile creatures, draconians, archons and luciferians. It is important to realize that negative entities of various types in a range of dimensions can imprint energetic tattoos onto people's bodies, within their houses and office's. Consequently, their vibration is clearly affected to a significant degree. Throughout the healing process we always look for any negative symbology and remove it.
 See Chapter 6 for more information.

Not all are dark but most are. Anunnaki and archons live on the earth in the fourth dimension, generally as undetectable energy fields, unless you have a gift to see through the veil. Draconians come from Planet X, or Nibiru. Luciferians are located 4.2 billion light years away yet can be down here in twenty-seven minutes via super highways, also known as black holes. These parasitic entities unilaterally practice deception on the human race as a means of control.

These beings can shift into this dimension, where they become detectable. Anunnaki have the ability to change into human form. If you think that someone is dark, or is a shape-shifting being, you can get him to identify himself with the following prayer, which will force them to show themselves.

As you say the prayer look into the person's face, where you might detect a translucent field around them revealing what they actually are. They can't hide. If the being is a reptile his eyes will change to reptilian eyes.

The first part of every prayer is always grounding.

Recognition Prayer

I am of God

I ground myself to the earth

Dear God, I command that you show

this person in their true form

through all space/time continuum

in every dimension

I thank You, God,

and send you my Unconditional Love

So Be It
Amen

If you see an opaque field of their actual reptilian shape, or if their eyes change, you can accept that they are reptilian and had best stay away from them. While there are good reptilian creatures out there, for the most part they are dark.

The other way to identify reptilian beings is to check by dowsing, or with a pendulum. Always proceed with the words, "In the name of God," before asking, "Is this person reptilian? Yes or no."The channel will be clear for 30 seconds because once you mention God any dark being will move away before returning. As mentioned before, Dark beings don't like the word "God," or anything angelic.

All beings are from God, the Omnipotent, but because of free will some become fallen souls and angels by choice. It is important not to be scared, but to adopt the tools that will help you identify who is a fallen angel or soul and who is of the light.

RULES TO LETTING GO

1. Concentrate on your gift and putting it to work. Think only about the creation of your work and infuse it with joy, not thought of monetary reward. If you even think you are creating something in order to pay a bill, you block the energy flow.

2. Have the faith to spend a little money to get a lot back. If you put money and energy out there they will come back to you a thousand fold.

3. Have the inner strength to get back out there again and again in order to maintain momentum.

4. Never think, "I'm broke." Instead, repeat when paying bills, "Is this all I have to pay?" Think and say throughout the course of the day, "I've got everything I need."

CHAPTER 2

Religions, Dogma & Fear

The Laws of God

Several years after leaving England I settled near my wife's home bordering the Ozark mountains in the Midwestern U.S., in a primarily white, Southern Baptist community. One day I entered a neighborhood gas station to get coffee, and holding the door open for a woman entering behind me, I struck up a light conversation as I typically do. The woman, who was African American, stared back at me with a shocked expression.

I reached the counter, and realizing I'd left my wallet in the car, headed back outside. When I returned, the woman stepped forward and stopped me from paying. She said, "I'm going to buy you that coffee, sir."

It was my turn to register shock as I asked why she would buy a complete stranger coffee. She answered, "I've been here for three months, and you're the first person to talk to me in any way."

I turned to the customers in the gas station, which was fairly full, dumfounded. "Isn't it time we concentrated on the teachings of Jesus?" I asked them. "Are we supposed to walk on the other side of the road when someone needs help?" Sheepish looks were exchanged. Excluding others is another a form of bullying. I realized then, that allegedly Christian communities still didn't understand the teachings of Jesus, and especially not the greatest teaching of all, that of Unconditional Love. Instead, religious organizations and their followers choose to focus on dogma and grasp watered-down teachings as the word of God, which are used as an excuse to create separation, unhappiness, and hate.

The bible we use today was created by the governmental system in charge at the time of its writing. It doesn't take a genius to realize that there is an inordinate amount of fear impregnated into the bible's words, meant to facilitate a system where followers donate their time and money to their chosen religious representatives in exchange for a place in heaven. In case you think I'm talking only about Christianity, rest assured that I address all organizations that put their creed in front of the Laws of God, which begin and end with Unconditional Love toward all living beings.

Heaven and Hell

There is no heaven or hell where God is concerned, instead, there is only Unconditional Love. We are here to love one another, full stop. Heaven and hell exists here on this planet, and you have the choice to live in either one. To choose heaven you need to be in a high vibrational state of Unconditional Love, Absolute Faith, and Peace. This energy is reflected outward to the surrounding community, where it is passed onward creating an ever-increasing ripple effect.

Living in heaven on earth means not worrying about the day-to-day trials that cross your life, and knowing instead, that divinity will always bless you. Living in heaven means fully letting go, accepting your divine purpose with absolutely no fear, and knowing that the Universal Creator, the God of All That Is, will take care of you and all life's necessities. The divine will provide all that you need to live a comfortable life.

I've found through my teachings that the act of letting go is one of the most difficult things for human beings to accomplish. Often it takes hitting rock bottom and experiencing hell on earth to fully let go. Rather than reach this point, step backward and give up fear. Fear is what creates hell on earth.

I see many people going to their place of worship and asking for forgiveness when they are not in a space to hand themselves over to God. For this you need to be in a state of Unconditional Love, peace and faith, where you forgive each circumstance and individual who may have wronged you in this life. Unconditional Forgiveness is the first step to obtaining absolute peace.

Forgiveness is the most powerful tool we have. I'll use the example of rape, which is epidemic in America. I've seen many, many rape victims. The key to initiating the healing process is Absolute Forgiveness. Very often we do a ceremony to release the energy of fear, hurt, anger, blame, or other emotions affecting the individual. We release these emotions to the universe and to God, allowing Him to take care of it, and allowing the victim to attain a state of Unconditional Love and tranquility. We'll go further into this in the healing chapters.

Christ Consciousness & Unconditional Love

When you are in a high vibrational state of "Christ Consciousness," no negative energies or entities can affect you. You will lead a completely blessed life. If you think about it, if God is Unconditional Love, then God has forgiven us down here for anything we do before we've done it. God never judges us. The life you lead is your journey and we have been put on earth to experience it in the way that we choose.

Earth is a testing ground where each individual possesses free will. To grow spiritually you have to experience the good things in life as well as the bad things. From these experiences we grow spiritually, learn, and move towards a higher vibrational level. The ultimate level is Christ Consciousness. Our avatars or ascended masters have come down with Christ Consciousness and are here to show us how to attain this level. The ascended masters are here at this time because we are currently experiencing the most important change the earth has ever gone through. All the ascended masters, Buddha, Jesus the Christ, Moses, Babaji, Enoch, the disciples, and others, are here right now to help us through this period.

The opposite of Christ Consciousness is low vibration. This dark energy is called hell on earth. Here you can spend your life being miserable, grumpy, depressed, and full of recriminations and blame. People spend time in this dark consciousness talking about other individuals behind their backs and condemning others instead of looking at themselves. How backward is that? People with lowered vibration need to take control over their own lives. Everything you experience you create. If you wallow in depression and grouchiness you create more of it. If your mind settles on lack, you won't be able to pay your bills. Your life becomes full of the negativity you create. It takes true inner strength to be able to leave behind the cauldron of misery and turn your life around. The first step is to approach every single experience you encounter as a blessed opportunity for spiritual growth and knowledge. Put a completely positive spin on everything you experience.

Sometimes, when something seemingly tragic happens, or some situation that's difficult to deal with arises, we don't see the blessings of the journey until later on when it's effect has a positive impact on your life. This is where faith comes in. Understand and believe that the situation will affect you positively.

Your True Path

I personally underwent a dramatic change several years ago when, in the process of going bankrupt, I lost my home and all remnants of the life I had known. I recall sitting in the middle of Manchester, England with two grocery bags of clothes representing all the possessions I had in the world. "Is this all I've got for my years of toil and sacrifice?" I asked God.

His reply was quite prominent: "It is the right time." I asked what He meant, and once again His reply was, "It's the right time, you will see." What a blessing it was, I soon agreed. All the third dimensional trappings of goods, Bentley's, houses, and trinkets had been taken from me. The loans on those things had also been removed, as well as my worry over paying off the debt and trying to keep up in the corporate race. I had been given an opportunity to completely change my life.

This blessed experience allowed me to focus on my true path and to utilize the gifts that God had given me. For each one of us has divine gifts. My gift showed itself not as painting, singing, or building things. It was healing. It is important for each of us to focus on our special talents, for doing so allows amazing things to happen. When you live in absolute faith you will find that the universe and God bless you many times over.

During this period of transforming from rags to spiritual richness, I experienced an epiphany. My newfound freedom afforded me the time to spend many hours meditating, and I discovered who I was in my previous lives transpiring over the past four thousand years, and received complete understanding as to why I was here. I was told about the part I have had since the universe was first created. I therefore asked God for His help in putting my life in this existence together so we could move forward on the spiritual journey. There is no such thing as coincidence, and incidents then coincided to bring my true partner, my soulmate, back into my life. I found her in Branson, Missouri, not by accident. I was spending time healing in Belize, when I helped a woman there free herself of a painful attachment to darkness. Upon her later visit to the States, she introduced me to a friend who brought another friend to dinner. When I saw this woman I immediately recognized her as the soul I had been with in the past. The bond we had was absolute, amazing, and it was divine. This oneness we had with each other lacked anger, fear, jealousy, and encompassed only love and absolute peace. The manifestation was complete.

Ginelle and I married. After we settled into the ministry I had a discussion with God and the universe about how it was their responsibility to take care of the bank account and cash flow, leaving me to focus on God's healing gifts. This incipient relationship with God has prospered, causing the ministry to flourish. My focus truly is on people, not on monetary reward. When your focus is on the good of humanity and of people rather than on monetary reward, the gifts bless you a million fold. This precept holds true across many religions and is well represented in Buddhism and Jesus' teachings.

During this time of setting up the ministry I believed that my path was to establish an interfaith church in Branson. One day as I was meditating, the true message came across loud and clear: *the church is within*. God told me to get out and be amongst people. A church is a mere building. It's what's inside that counts. So Ginelle and I went out and met people, which has brought us to today. Although neither of us had money we managed to settle the ministry through faith.

I want to repeat, when I went bankrupt all the fear of bills disappeared. I had to truly let go of everything for my life to change. Letting go, I remind you, is having absolutely no fear of anything at all, and knowing that God protects you.

Jesus, Melchizedek Beings, and Creator Gods

Jesus the Christ, is Jesus of the Christ Consciousness. He was a Melchizedek Being who came down here to teach people about living in Unconditional Love and in peaceful tranquility. He did not come to judge people, yet He was always there to forgive. If you look back at his teachings you'll find they are all about forgiveness. Never judge people as sinners. Only the person who has never done wrong in his life can cast the first stone. Remember, life is a journey that's about learning. If you focus on the teachings of Jesus and not on the dogma, your spiritual growth will be incredible. The same teachings have been told to us by Buddha, Sai Baba, and all the ascended masters. No matter what you call Him, whether it's Yahweh, Elohim, The Big Cheese, Allah, All That Is—whatever amazing force God is, He loves us unconditionally. I was invited once to a bible class, and the first thing they said was "it says in the bible we are all sinners." My reply was, if we are created in the image of God and we are all sinners, then what does that make God? At that point a kerfuffle started until I went on to say, "If we are created in the image of God, we are each unconditional loving beings in a third dimensional school learning our spiritual growth. We have come back many times to experience this journey which brings us closer to Christ Consciousness."

It is important when reading any religious text that you are guided with your true gut feeling, the inner knowing of whether or not the teachings are correct. The governmental systems have always been in place to manipulate the people and keep them in a fearful state. The journey we're pursuing down here, which can cover many thousands of lifetimes, is a journey of free will. If you don't attain the Christ Consciousness in your lifetime you will be sent back to the third dimensional classroom on earth again and again, until eventually reaching that high vibrational state. Only you can decide what is right and wrong, and to prevent things from manipulating you. As I travel around I see huge religious organizations that have become corporate monetary machines and not organizations of Unconditional Love. Dogma is pushed by the third dimensional control systems which uses scripture as a fear mechanism, frightening and controlling people, and causing them to part with income as a means of getting into heaven. This flatly fails, as explained earlier. You, me—we are all sinners until we truly give to others. True giving comes from the heart in its many forms, and has no expectation of getting anything back. Dogma, and anything else that frightens you, bears a closer look. Use your gut feelings to determine whether it is right or wrong. If we focus on the teachings of Jesus, Sai Baba, and the other ascended masters, we will find ourselves in a much better place, then if we follow those institutions secretly guided by money and control.

The true journey of Jesus has been sadly obscured. Jesus was born in Nazara, an ancient town in Egypt. Bethlehem didn't exist in the time of Christ, but came about ninety years later. If you ask a Vatican cardinal, he will admit that the bible is not wholly correct. Jesus was caught by the Romans and put on the cross. The Romans believed that after three days the soul leaves the body, and so concluding that he was clinically dead, they allowed Jesus to be taken from the cross and directed his people never to return. Mary Magdalene and others transported Jesus to France and settled in a town called Tarot, where they were allowed to grow spiritually. They developed the tarot cards, and received their own divine answers. Tarot cards have since been tampered with. The tarot we see today are not the ancient tools of holy divination Jesus and Mary created. The original ancient tarot, not the ones which have been adulterated, contained a vibration which allowed you to get all the answers you desired, directly from God.

The Resurrection, as we have been told the story, is figurative. His consciousness expanded and Jesus escaped the system of control and returned to a place of Unconditional Love. He healed people and lived out his life until His work was done. His purpose completed, he ascended. Melchizedek beings never die; they ascend and the body disappears. There is nothing to bury.

The life of Jesus will be explored more fully in the future.

Creator Gods genetically spliced human beings from their own selves and sent humans down here, to earth. They are in charge of the human being *soul recycling process*, which involves sending us here to attain spiritual growth until reaching Christ Consciousness. Melchizedek beings are from the ultimate dimension and sit with God of the Universe. The Creator Gods agreed with the Galactic Federation and God of the Universe to create a human race that could feel emotions and obtain spiritual growth while learning Absolute Faith.

Getting Into the Godspace

The concept of reincarnation was eliminated from the bible, although it was dressed up as heaven or hell, or as "going to the God realm." What this means is that when you reach the heaven part of experience, you are completing your journey. The hell part is becoming mired in the negativity that prevents you from completing your journey. This wisdom has been eliminated from the bible as an additional measure of control. Governmental systems don't want people to know they are in charge of their own destinies. If we don't want to come back to the hell, we must get into the Godspace with Absolute Faith. Fear kills faith. Release and let go of all fear and strive for a peaceful, loving state. This does not mean to separate yourself from the wrong around you, but rather, to forgive from a place of peace and tranquility.

I get many fearful emails about things going on in the world. Clearly, if there was universal Unconditional Love and peace there would be no war. Send all situations Unconditional Love. If enough people do this, the situation will collapse. Your actions can change the world. Simply by achieving Christ Consciousness you are uplifting the vibration of this third dimensional universe. It's important to focus on doing your part. If millions of people do this, the whole world will change.

Even though our food is tampered with, if you create the reality that it won't harm you and instead will nourish you, and do this with Absolute Faith in God, then the toxins won't touch you (see the *Food Prayer*). Take a step away from fearful things and be at peace. Going further into that, stop buying the products of companies that tamper with our food and engage in illicit practices. Don't allow anger to come in. If you stop buying their products these corporations will go out of business. They only way to approach every situation is with Unconditional Love and Peace.

Healing in God's Name

I've seen various healers invoking the Lord's name when healing, yet their patients remain ill. It's important to understand the underlying factors of divine healing. It's not just talk, or invoking God's name that has an effect, but rather, the individual changing his life for the better. Some of us are taught to believe that if you ignore the dark side it will go away. The truth is the opposite. The dark forces surrounding you will keep manipulating you until you stop them from affecting you, and block their negative energetic frequencies from your life. To do so you must step outside third dimensional thinking and reject its so-called misery. It takes great faith and courage to be able to do this. Removing the blinders and stepping into the place of Absolute Faith takes inner peace, letting go, and freeing yourself of the manipulation of 3D substances, whether they be in the form of toxic foods, mind-altering substances, pharmaceuticals, or blindly following dogma and rhetoric through subliminal mind control.

Starseeds and Receiving Your Gifts

If you are a starseed and not on the right path, very often God will remove things from your life, causing you to hit rock bottom. This is a means of getting you to reevaluate and change your world. For others who are already on the journey, following your path is a matter of free will. Some people don't ever step out of the box and attain Christ Consciousness. If so, it isn't their journey to do so. You should never be frustrated by things other people are, or are not, attaining. Accept the journey of others for what it is, and know your journey is truly just about you. Having made the shift I can say with certainty that doing so allows God's bounty to bless you every day. It's a blessing that comes without ego, knowing you are on the right path and doing something to uplift humanity.

Normally, starseeds have interesting gifts; a high level of intuition, the ability to see inter-dimensional spirits, and a very loving spirit, even though they may be manipulated. They know they are different. In our classes on discovering our gifts, we generally look at what you've been doing for the last four thousand years, which is a rehearsal for what you are here to do now. We conduct a regression to find out which starseed race you're from, and connect to the race through portals in their dimension. Most starseed races are from the fifth dimension. There are thousands of starseeds on the planet right now. Some have been stifled, misled, shut down, stuffed full of entities, and more. There are many ways to shut down a starseed, from fear and anger, to the chemicals in our food and the fluoride in our toothpaste, which close the pineal down. There have never been as many starseeds as there are on this planet today. The people in control know who they are and are trying to block their gifts. Being of high vibration helps immensely.

The way to find out where you are from is as follows. Use your intuition and ask: *Am I Pleiadian? Arcturian? Sumerian? Atlantarian? Andromedan?*

Wherever you're from, ask God to open a portal to that dimension and to put the other end of the portal around you. Meditate through that dimension, asking to receive information. Your starseed family will download the information and your gifts as you connect to them. Ask God to send energy to your pineal to break down the crystallization. The pineal is the seat of our connection to the higher universe.

A healing to open the pineal gland can be found on our YouTube channel, accessed through the Macklin Ministries website at:

WWW.CHRISTOPHERMACKLINMINISTRIES.COM

Turning Your Life Around

The opposite of Christ Consciousness is low vibration. This dark energy is called hell on earth, and here you can spend your life being miserable, grumpy, depressed, and full of recriminations and blame. Everything you experience you create. If you wallow in depression and grouchiness you create more of it. If your mind settles on lack, you won't be able to pay your bills.

Put a positive spin on everything in your life. Your life becomes full of the positivity you create. It takes true inner strength to be able to turn your life around.

Remember, every single experience you encounter is a blessed opportunity for spiritual growth and knowledge.

Chapter 3

The Importance of Meridians, Energy and High Vibration

Take a good look at a Chinese medicine diagram and note the body's twelve main meridian paths. While these lines may look like straight pathways, they are in fact highly interconnected. When healing someone's liver the individual might feel sensation in the bottom of their foot, for example, because that meridian pathway is being triggered, generating phantom feelings elsewhere in the body. What people don't always realize is that surgical operations disconnect the meridian energy paths to connected areas and block the energy flow to the organs located there. It becomes more difficult for the body to heal when it's meridian flow is blocked due to the pathways being severed. When scar tissue forms, the meridians become further blocked. Once, a young female patient came to me who had undergone an operation to correct something in her abdomen. She was embarrassed by the scar, and although the operation had occurred sometime previously, she was still experiencing pain. Once we reconnected the pathways through the operative area and re-established meridian flow, then removed the scar tissue, the scar as well as the pain vanished. In my opinion, surgery should always be a last resort. It addresses the symptoms only and never the real cause, while its effects can cause untold lasting damage.

Body piercings and tattoos also sever the meridian pathways and cause issues to arise within the body, now or in the future. Anything that can potentially block meridian flow is not recommended.

Energy Healing

Einstein said, "Energy can never be destroyed; it only changes form." I like to say, "While energy can be transposed into different areas, it can never be created or destroyed. It is always there."

The first question people generally ask when coming to me for a healing is, "What exactly is divine healing?" My answer has always been, "If you listen to an orchestra, you will experience many different facets of sound—violin, oboe, kettle drum, harp—which together, form a complete ensemble."

The correlation to divine healing is that different facets of healing are used in combination to create the complete healing effect. Divine healing is not simply energy healing. Reiki, as mentioned earlier, was once effective, but during the past ten to twenty years the universal life force energy has dropped, rendering Reiki mostly ineffective. Energy workers who are tapping into third dimensional universal life force energy are simply not doing the job. They must tap into the fifth dimension, and because that dimension has not yet arrived; it must be accessed through a portal.

The difference between divine healing and energy healing is that divine healing addresses the actions of inter-dimensional entities, transmissional frequencies, and Nano-technology, and their negative physical, emotional, and spiritual effects on individuals. Divine healing utilizes the help of angelic beings, Melchizedek beings, inter-dimensional tachyon energy, and the Unconditional Love of God Energy to implement a wide variety of modalities, which in combination bring about complete healing. These modalities will soon be explained.

God of The Universe

The primary energy I use is that of God of The Universe in the ultimate dimension. It is important for healers to tap into the dimensional energy of their starseed family for the healing work to be the most effective.

Energy alone doesn't heal, although it helps alleviate things like pain. For example, if you have an entity over one knee causing blockages and creating arthritis, you can send energy there which will heal the pain, but the arthritis still remains. It's important to utilize different facets of healing to break down the calcification and therefore completely heal the knee.

Very often people ask me who God is, or who I perceive to be God.

God of the Universe can be perceived in whatever form you believe in—whether it be Elohim, Yahweh, Allah, The Universal Spirit, God, the Creator—but God of the Universe is all that is. I sometime call him "the Big Cheese in the Sky." I tell people that my wife is the second biggest cheese in the sky, in case they are ready for a laugh.

Vibration and Negative Attachments

One of the fundamental issues to address before conducting any healing is to access an individual's vibration. If the person has a disease of any type it means his vibration has dropped too low. Before we can move forward with healing it's critical to raise his vibration back to a high level using high-vibration inter-dimensional energy, and to remove toxins. The next thing I do is heal any negative energies or attachments within the body that are causing meridian blockages. These entities normally come from the first, second or fourth dimension. In those dimensions the entities have bodies, but appear in this dimension as an esoteric spirit of low vibration.

These inter-dimensional entities are called *IDE's*, and are of extremely low vibration. It bears mentioning that all entities are created by God, but have free will within their dimension, and have become fallen angels of low energy and greed.

The IDE's currently causing the most severe problems are generally snake beings from the 2nd dimension, and draconians, archons and anunnaki from the 4th dimension. To remove these energies the healer must be in a high vibrational state himself, or these entities will enter his body and make him as sick or sicker than the person being healed. To remove each IDE, I grab it's esoteric energy and pull it out of the patient's body.

How do IDE's enter your body in the first place? The root cause is normally a significant emotional or toxic issue occurring within the body. The emotional issue might be caused by the death of someone close, suicide within the family, divorce, or fallout from other emotionally taxing events. Due to emotional stress the vibration of your body drops. The negative entities around us love a negative energy party, and are able to get into your body at these times because their vibration is also low. This similar energy allows them to slip into your body with ease. The draconians and anunnaki, particualarly, like to sit within the abdomen, attach themselves to the lower back just above the sacrum, and manipulate the person by sending them negative thoughts through the spinal column. These thoughts are always *you thoughts*, such as "You are no good;" You will never succeed;" "You are fat," "ugly," "stupid," and so on. It is important to recognize *you thoughts* when you are feeling depressed, and to block them out.

Cause and Effect

Depending upon where the IDE, or entity, sits, whether its on the right or center of the abdomen, for example, it will drop the vibration of the organs they are sitting over, causing that organ or section of the body to become semi-paralyzed. This can cause many issues. If the IDE sits over the liver, the liver will stop functioning properly and won't process the toxins in the body. Therefore you will gain weight and get a heavy head, or toxic headaches. When the liver drops below 20% functionality, there are so many toxins in the body that they attack the platelets and bone marrow. This is how leukemia arises.

If the IDE is sitting more to the left, it can cause problems within the gastric tract. The gastric tract then becomes semi-paralyzed and fails to digest food in the correct position within the intestine, causing acid reflux, colonic issues, or poor absorption of nutrients.

If the entity sits over the pancreas, it drops the vibration of the pancreas causing diabetes.

If any affected area is not rectified, over a period of time you will find that fungal infections begin to manifest, eventually turning into cancer tumors.

If an entity sits low in the abdomen it can cause endometriosis in the womb lining, fibroids, the prostrate, or issues with the ovaries such as ovarian cysts. Doctors in the 3rd dimension don't understand the causes behind these issues and in female cases generally prescribe radical hysterectomies. This is not getting rid of the cause, it is exchanging one set of symptoms for another.

In other parts of the body, like the throat or lungs, a drop in vibrational energy can cause fungal infections and cancer to arise. In the case of fibromyalgia, defined by the medical community as possessing nine out of twenty-one symptoms ranging from headaches, lower back pain, muscle aches, and depression, entities sitting within the body are causing blockages and paralyzing organs, creating the symptoms.

If you think about it, a low vibrational entity in the lower part of the body is going to block the meridian flow stemming out from where that entity is. Some individuals only get arthritis in the right hand, elbow, or knee, and not in the left. Doctors attribute arthritis to old age, which in my opinion is ridiculous. It's worth asking the doctor why you are getting arthritis in the right hand, when your right and left hand are both the same age. I've experienced that when people get arthritis in the right hand and elbow, for example, it's because they have an attachment in the form of an inter-dimensional entity sitting within the shoulder blocking the meridian flow down the right side. The body needs energy flow as much as it needs blood flow. The body needs balance. If you have no energy flow in a particular area, the bones will start calcifying.

On the other hand, if your body is high vibration and you have complete meridian flow through your pathways, and if you are free of toxins, you will never get sick. There really are only a few causes of disease: toxicity; DNA issues; emotional issues; blocked meridian flow from trauma or surgery; or transmissional frequencies, all giving rise to IDE's. All damage to the body needs to be addressed in order for the body to be 100% healed.

Brain tumors, for instance, can be caused by ammonia and other toxins in the brain because the liver vibration has dropped and is failing to process the toxins within the body. Or, it may be caused by an inter-dimensional entity sitting within the individual's head.

We've found that one hundred percent of breast cancer, has been caused by a second dimensional being within the breast blocking its meridian structure. With no meridian energy through the pathways, fungal infections within the breast start manifesting and eventually develop into tumors.

Blindness can be caused by blood sugar issues, cataracts, deterioration of the eye membrane and more, all brought about by meridian blockages.

Heart and lungs are also affected by negative entities and meridian blockages. With a drop in vibration, the fungal infections can turn into tumors.

There are a variety of DNA issues that can cause disease. They can come from birth defects or from toxins through food or environment, such as EMF's or chemtrails, which change our DNA and cause disease. We'll explain later how these and all issues are corrected.

It's important to reinforce that emotional issues of any type are correlated to dropping the body vibration, therefore allowing low vibration inter-dimensional entities to get into the body.

Radionics

When people use radionic machines like biomodulators, supposedly to help heal, it is important to understand that they can not duplicate the spectral density of healing energy, for it is way too complex .

When using these machines it is essential that the operators are protected. If not, these machines can transmit esoteric spirits and negative vibrational compounds to the patient being healed.

Radionic machines can make you sicker. If you decide to use them anyway, it's important to protect these machines with the the following prayer:

Esoteric Pyramid Prayer of Protection

I am of God

I ground myself to the Earth

I command You, God, to remove all the radionic manipulation from this machine that is not for my highest good

through the space/time continuum in every dimension

I bring all the people involved in this manipulation, no matter how remote

In every dimension, before You, God, for justice in only the way you know how.

I release them to You with Unconditional Love and Forgiveness

I thank You, God, and send you my Unconditional Love

So Be It
Amen

Tachyon Energy and The Time-Space Continuum Change

Tachyon energy is synonymous with changing the time-space continuum and is a very unique form of energy. The tachyon energy you may be hearing about these days on the internet and in movies, is very different from what I am referring to. The tachyon energy used for divine healing comes from the ultimate dimension, and allows me to revert the body to a previous time and bring it forward on a different timeline. This methodology has an extremely high impact on the body and tends to tire people out during the healing cycle. This energy is not normally used for illnesses, but at times when trauma has taken place, like a car crash, when you can define a specific time when the body was completely functional and intact. We raise the vibration of a person's body and then apply inter-dimensional tachyon energy to the part of the body that's been affected by the trauma. This energy feels very different within the body. When the whole body is high enough or "tachyonized," we can then step back in time, thus changing the space time continuum of that part of the body, to a time when it was completely functional before the trauma happened. We then bring that part of the body back on a new timeline and reintegrate it back into the body so there is no time-space shift.

Incidentally, when I say "we" I refer to "the team," which consists of God of the Universe, and the Melchizedek Beings and those from the Angelic Realm who participate in the healings. I don't take responsibility for the healings, but consider myself a facilitator, blessed with the gift to help people heal. I am, and always will be, a humble servant of God.

There is a time lag between the start of the manifestation and its completion. Sometimes it takes up to four or five days for the manifestation to complete. The person receiving this form of healing will feel almost paralyzed while this manifestation is taking place. Again, this is not normally used for people with a major illness, but for issues caused by something concrete, like trauma. I am guided by the angelic realm as to when to use this modality. We have found, however, that tachyon energy is useful for treating Lyme disease.

Because the space time continuum changes, when applied to Lyme, it destroys the borrelia with no die-off. We will share more about this further on.

Tachyon Healing Examples

I had a female patient who had been in a car crash two years earlier which left her with major spine issues, including a cracked vertebrae and severely damaged discs. She was taken to the hospital and because her vibration had dropped after the trauma, she had entities within her. We removed these and revibrated her body. It took a few healing sessions to get her vibrational energy high enough to begin healing. Once we did this, we applied tachyon energy to her entire spine. We then took her back in time, changed the space-time continuum of the spine, brought the spine back on a new timeline and reintegrated it into her body. This rendered the patient almost incapacitated until the manifestation was complete. When it was finished, she arose and her spine was completely healed.

An older man came to me who was suffering from major diabetes. His blood sugar level was 600. Once we removed the entity and revibrated the pancreas, we began work on his blindness, for his eyes had grown milky and he couldn't see beyond a foot in front of him. We tachyonized his eyes, took him back to a time when his eyes were fully functional, in his case 1982, and brought his eyes back on a new timeline. Then we reintegrated them into his body, so that there was no time-phase shift between his eyes and the timeline of his body. Within 24 hours his eyes were no longer milky and he was back to normal.

Walk-Ins and Soul Contracts

When I took the gentleman with diabetes back in time I was attempting to get back to 1976, but I found his timeline stopped in 1982. I tried again and again to get back to 1976, but the timeline remained firm at 1982. I asked God why this was. He told me it was because my patient was a walk-in, and that his soul was replaced in 1982.

There are a number of gifted people down here who have agreed in a soul contract to allow a soul replacement to enter their body after they have lived a certain amount of time in this third dimension. This means that one soul remains within the body while the other is attached, so that the souls run parallel and both receive the experience of this lifetime. The parallel soul experiences all the things that are happening here, but without the pain, emotion and the trauma.

At a particular point in time the souls are swapped over, and the new soul enters the body while the soul that's been here up to this time goes back to the God Realm. The new soul will see the body back to its ultimate conclusion.

This happens because it is very difficult to live on this earth and to utilize one's gifts in light of the negativity that's occurring here. A walk-in allows the new soul to move forward with the gifts and to accomplish the things you are supposed to be doing.

When a walk-in steps in, a slight change may be perceived by those around you, but not a radical enough difference for them to notice the change.

The Thinning Veil and Cellular Energy

Because the veil is currently thinning between third and fifth dimensions, esoteric transference is occurring with increasing frequency. To explain further, esoteric transference is when things that have happened in past lives have been carried over to the present. For example, if you'd been killed by a dagger in a previous lifetime, you might find some of its symptoms or effects slipping through the veil. You might experience terrible pain where the dagger hit, because the energy field is still within your body. Or you might be still experiencing the effects of a previous illness, like cancer. To address this we remove the old energy field and reconnect the body's meridian pathways so they function correctly, thus allowing normal energy flow down the body.

Use your gut instinct to ascertain whether you are experiencing esoteric transference
and ask your higher consciousness, or God, whether you have cellular energy within your body. If you get a "yes," then you need to release it.

To release this cellular energy the past life prayer needs to be said three or nine times, as these numbers are sacred within the sacred geometry. This will be addressed fully in future books, but briefly, sacred geometry is a number system based on the Fibonacci series and pyramid structures.

Each time you say the prayer you should feel some sort of release within the body. It is important to say every prayer with absolute authority.

Prayer to Release Any Cellular Memory or Esoteric Transference From Past Life

Dear God

I come before you now for forgiveness

for anything I have done

in any past life to infinitum

through all space/time continuum

in every dimension

that has been brought back into this lifetime

and is affecting me now

I release it all to You, God,
with Unconditional Love

I thank You, God,

and send you my Unconditional Love

So Be It
Amen

You can say it to yourself or aloud, but it's important to feel a spiritual shiver each time you do so, indicating that the prayer is being activated. If you don't feel the shiver say it again until you do. As I've come to know, God likes a little bit of feistiness.

This prayer will release all the embossed cellular energy from your body. If you don't feel that it's been released, then say the prayer nine times, in three lots of three over three days to allow time for your body to release the cellular energy.

Human Transcendence

It's interesting to note that lightening appears very different nowadays than it has in the past. This is because the thinning veil is creating inter-dimensional static between the fifth and the third dimensions. How can you recognize this? When lightening strikes create a spider-web type matrix of static, appearing like a grid instead of a flash, it is actually inter-dimensional static in the form of sacred geometry.

Why is the veil so thin? Because we are in the process of transcending to the fifth dimension. As we grow closer the electrostatic differences between the dimensions becomes more prominent. If you put a pole next to a high tension wire, the electricity between the two items will arc. This is the same principle as inter-dimensional static. As the two dimensions near each other the electricity increases and grows visible.

This transcendence into the 5th dimension is a two dimensional shift, not a one dimensional shift. We are leaping over the fourth dimension, where negative entities exist, to the fifth dimension. This transcendence has been in place for eons and is occurring because too much darkness has welled up here in the third dimension. God of the Universe has decided to switch to the fifth dimension in order to rid us of the darkness.

Many people were expecting this change to occur on the 21st of December 2012, as predicted by the Mayans. That change is still due to happen, and strangely enough, still on that date. This is because the date has not yet arrived due to the fact that the space time continuum has been manipulated by the dark forces. The space time continuum is being manipulated as we speak, and it is my belief that transcendence will happen at the latest by March 2015.

The arrival of that date is not changeable because the *universal time markers* have been stretched. This is a complex topic that we'll talk about it in further depth later on and in other books.

Explanations of a full range of illnesses and healing modalities follow.

How to Tell if You are Loving Unconditionally and in Alignment

1. You feel at peace, with no stress or worry

2. You have no negative thoughts

3. You laugh all the time

4. You are excited and positive about everything

5. You care for the welfare of strangers as much as you do for yourself

Chapter 4

Causes of Illness and How to Heal Them

When people are being healed, it's very important that the healer uses his spiritual gifts to understand the causes behind the issue, how they manifested and what additional external issues are affecting the individual now. As mentioned before, there are a variety of factors that can cause the body to have disease, including emotions, toxins, viruses, stealth pathogens, transmissional frequencies, DNA defects, esoteric transference and cellular memory. These things can affect the body spiritually, physically and emotionally. Therefore, when healing, all three areas need to be addressed. If the cause is not removed the symptoms reappear. For this reason I first look at identifying the cause.

Identifying the Cause

Whether the cause is emotional, physical or spiritual, I always ask the angelic realm to show me what trauma allowed the manifestation of disease within the individual's body. Normally, they show me video of that trauma. It is important then, to address that trauma by giving the person being healed unconditional forgiveness and Unconditional Love. Sending the same to the person or situation responsible for the trauma, is equally as important. If toxins are at fault, we remove them by switching them out via the space time continuum through the portal, and rebalancing the autoimmune system. If you don't rebalance the autoimmune system, it can cause inflammation because it still behaves as if the toxin is there. People think divine healing is simple, but it's quite complicated. It's like being a doctor, in a way. Each situation is different, but there are generalities that are the same for most. We'll go further into deep traumas caused by things like rape, past karma, and cancers, a bit later.

Karmic Lessons and Forgiveness

When you come into this lifetime in this 3D world, your karma is reset. As a baby, you have come here with no karma whatsoever. You create your karma on your life's journey. If you do something very bad then sometimes the Creator Gods will bring you back to them, because you are not learning in this lifetime. Suffering is part of our lifetime journey, for it is how we learn to forgive. If you are not learning you are likely to acquire some disease because of negativity or low vibration, and go back to the Creator Gods. They will allow you to understand the mistakes you are making then send you back in another lifetime to learn again.

It's important when healing to ask God and the angelic realm whether or not you, as the person being healed, are on a karmic lesson. If the answer is "yes," then it's important to find out if you're in a place to ask God for forgiveness. If you did a wrong thing like kill someone, for instance, if you ask God for forgiveness and truly feel it, then your karma will be reset. If you don't truly feel repentance, then you will be taken back through the soul recycling process and begin again.

If someone has wronged you in an extreme way, and they are still alive, you must release them to God with Unconditional Love and forgiveness and ask God to take care of the karma. To do this we have a simple prayer:

Prayer to Release Karma

I am of God

I ground myself to the earth

Dear God, I realize this person (name)

has wronged me and it is not for me to judge

him/her in any way,

through all space/time continuum
in every dimension

Dear God, I bring this person before you

for justice in only the way you know how.

And I release him/her to you

with Unconditional Love and Forgiveness

I thank you, God,

and send you my Unconditional Love

So Be It
Amen

When the individual is released to God, the energy from your heart chakra is sent out into the universe. This releases the emotional issues that have been blocking your life as well.

If the person who has wronged you has passed, the karma can be reset in a different way. In this instance we ask permission from God to bring the soul back for forgiveness. This can only be done if the patient is in the right space to allow forgiveness to occur. Sometimes it can take a few sessions to get in the right space. You have to have an overwhelming knowing that the forgiveness is there in your heart. When we do a session of forgiveness, we feel the transgressor's soul come into the room. He's normally allowed five minutes to express all the emotions surrounding the past wrongdoing. This occurs on an esoteric level. We then get the patient to give the soul Unconditional Love and forgiveness. This releases the soul from the karma and allows the soul to move on to the next lifetime or wherever it's meant to go, in order to spiritually move on. The person down here who's been wronged can then move along, for the emotion that's been blocking his life has been released.

Esoteric Transference and Cellular Memory

People think they come down here with "bad" karma because they've got issues from past lives, when in fact that's not the case. If you have issues with your body arising from the past lives, it is because the energy from that lifetime has accidentally gotten through the veil that separates dimensions and is affecting your energy now. This can be cellular memory in the lower back causing back issues, or it can be phantom pain throughout your abdomen because you were killed by a sword in a former life and that sword's energy field has accidentally slipped through the veil. It's important to ascertain what has slipped through the field and to release it, whether it's the esoteric field or cellular memory. Related issues will disappear once the area has been revibrated. Esoteric transference is energy transference embossed on the soul that manifests in the body as an energy field. Cellular memory is deeply embossed, low-vibrational energy at cellular level which is "stuck" and needs to be released.

Why is the veil thin? Because we are transcending to the fifth dimension where the Creator Gods are.

You decide to be born to a particular parent. If there are defects in your DNA, you have chosen to come into the lifetime and experience them. This is not karma, this is choice. When you pass, you experience the emotions of the people you have affected while you were alive and learn from this. You then decide what you want to focus on in the next lifetime for your spiritual growth. Karma is created by you, not imposed upon you. You do not retain karma from past lives, but you may have esoteric transference, a mistake that's transpired because the veil is too thin. You are perfect when you enter the body.

DNA

People can be born with genetic defects caused by toxins within the mother, frequencies, or negative inter-dimensional manipulations which manifest into disease. This includes Parkinson's, Cystic Fibrosis, and all genetic diseases. Correcting DNA defects requires revibrating the person's body, bringing it to a heightened vibration, and removing all negative entities and meridian blockages. Once the individual's vibration has achieved a high enough level, we can invoke a DNA change. This is a manifestation that runs throughout the body starting from the sacral point, which is where life began and is also the center of the merkaba field. Genetic manifestation takes, normally, between four and six weeks and renders the person unstable during this time and sort of bipolar, where they feel happy one minute and may be crying the next. This disorientation is temporary, and I prepare people for it by letting them know we are changing their whole being. The manifestation starts in the sacral point in the cells, then manifests outward throughout the body. After the manifestation completes in four to six weeks, the genetic condition disappears.

Sometimes the genetic defect is an entity-driven defect from this dimension, put in place by manipulation. Sometimes whole families suffer from chronic issues like depression, for example, because of entities. Because the behavior connections in a bloodline can go back many generations to one person who had a toxin or who was manipulated, it can be passed down, feathering out among subsequent generations

Transmissional Frequencies

Transmissional frequencies are manmade emissions of low or high frequencies within the air space—such as those generated by cell towers, computers, wireless devices, cell phones, tablets, smart phones, radio, television, or radionic machines— whether it be low frequencies of hertz (Hz) or kilohertz (kHz), or high satellite frequencies of terahertz (THz). It's no wonder there's so much illness, with the amount of transmissional frequencies we experience on a second-by-second basis.

Toxins, Viruses and Stealth Pathogens

Toxins are rife in this dimension. They exist in our food, in our water, and in the air, and they are radically affecting people's bodies. Toxins like heavy metals poison us through our food supply, through chemtrails, and our teeth. Toxins are low vibrational and drop the vibration of the body. Toxins can be eradicated. They can be switched out through the space time continuum into a different dimension and the body can be revibrated to get its vibration up to the higher consciousness level.

There are a variety of viruses, but they cannot live in a high vibrational body. If you are sick then your vibration is not where it should be. Practice meditation, yoga, forgiveness, positive thinking, and living without fear, anger or recriminations. Switch off the TV. Do not take vaccines. Doctors give us low vibrational toxins in the form of pills that make things worse. Try to remain on an organic, non-GMO, medicine-free diet. In the prayer chapter a prayer is given to revibrate anything that you might ingest. I think it's fair to say that in a high vibrational world, medicines and vaccines are completely unnecessary. These things that have been drummed into our consciousness as effective, they aren't. In a high vibrational world they are acknowledged as unnecessary, and no longer harm us. We need to take a more childlike approach to life, where we are unconditional loving beings, having fun, in inner peace and happiness. All of this correlates to a high vibration and will allow you to flourish. Don't take fear into your heart chakra, including fear of death or dire prognoses for illnesses. No illness is a death sentence. What it is, is a manifestation of an issue you must address and eradicate. Then the illness will disappear. Remember from the first chapter, that if someone points a gun at your chest and is squeezing the trigger you can manifest your own death or a new reality, with absolute faith where you don't die.

The chemtrails that pollute the skies with crisscrossing plumes of smoke, are delivering a full supply of toxins, including aluminum, barium, borrelia, strontium and Nano-particles. When these particles come into contact with skin they sink in and start growing within the body. These pathogens and Nano particles replicate exponentially throughout the body, creating a web-like matrix that can transmit and receive frequencies like a biological computer. Additionally, the stealth pathogens and Nano particles block the meridian structure completely. We have a way of dealing with these toxins, utilizing the time space continuum.

You can't send people with borrelia (Lyme disease), for instance, high volumes of normal energy, because the toxic die-off can be so extreme as to create anaphylactic shock. Instead, in instances like Lyme we rebalance energies and switch out the toxins in space and time to balance the body with no die-off. We have a protocol for Lyme which uses tachyon energy in very high doses to change the complete molecular structure of the borrelia, thus rendering it harmless to the body. This technique is proving an amazing success and completely eliminates Lyme from the body.

We use the same tachyon energy technique on Morgellons disease. The tachyon energy destroys the Nano particles creating the disease, and changes their molecular structure to render them inactive. Morgellons, which is not officially recognized as a disease by the medical community, gives rise to symptoms that include plastic balls, carbon fibers and biofilm being released through the skin. It is systematic and debilitating, not to mention terrifying to see foreign, spidery objects exit through your skin, some of which are moving of their own accord and are mechanical in nature.

Agent Orange is similar in nature to Morgellons, as is borrelia and HIV. The toxins creating these diseases consist of spirochetes, a stealth pathogen. Stealth pathogens in these instances possess an unusual molecular structure and the unique ability to completely bypass the human immune system.

The degree in which individuals are effected by Morgellons is dependent upon their genetics. Everyone has Morgellons particles within them due to unavoidable exposure via chemtrails and other environmental toxins. The strength of your genetics determines whether Morgellons will develop. Those who experience spider-type creatures, for instance, possess a weakened Chromosome 53. We have had success in healing this disease, but it is a time-consuming and in-depth process. Morgellons can be activated by military frequencies and some people experience excruciating pain when these frequencies are switched on. These frequencies are transmitted by satellite in the terahertz range 10 to the 12th THz. This is yet another reason to keep your vibration up. No illness can live in a high vibrational body, even borrelia and the Nano toxins associated with Morgellons. Low vibration changes your DNA. If you experience any of these symptoms you need to get your vibration up and likely, you need to change out your DNA. Lyme disease and Morgellons travel together. If you have Morgellons you definitely have Lyme disease, but you can have Lyme without Morgellons. Again, this depends upon your DNA, or genetic make-up.

Mass healings are in place now and future training sessions are planned to try and address these and other growing health issues all over the world, as quickly as possible.

How the Modalities Work

Inter-dimensional energy is drawn through portals into this dimension in order to facilitate healing. This portal opens to the higher dimension that the healer is drawing energy from, and opened at the other end around the person being healed, and closing beneath him so that he fits completely within the portal. This, on its own will change the space time continuum. I've had many reports that the hour-long healing session only felt like five minutes to the patient. This is because there is no time within a portal.

Using the angelic realm from the higher dimension, we are utilizing an energy with a much higher vibration that is sent down the body to revibrate its molecular structure and allowing the person to ascend to a much higher vibration, one that is close to Christ Consciousness.

Revibrating someone's body once doesn't get them completely to the Christ Consciousness, or the God Space; it can take several sessions for the body vibration to change. It's like a staircase. If you revibrate once it takes them up four steps. Allowing for three days between sessions, they'll drop back a step. We'll revibrate them again and they'll ascend four more steps and drop back one, until we reach to the top of the staircase. It is only then that the body reaches Christ Consciousness, located at the top of the staircase.

To maintain the vibration, it's essential to focus on positive thinking between sessions, and to not let anyone influence you negatively, in any way. This includes staying away from energy vampires, the people who literally suck your energy and lower your vibration by speaking or doing things to bring down your life force. Meditation, yoga, and creative endeavors help keep your vibration high.

Entity Clearing

Jesus called them demonic entities; I call them fallen souls and fallen angels. As mentioned earlier, entities can get into the body if your energy level has dropped significantly through some turbulence in your life, be it emotional in nature, due to transmissional frequencies, or toxins. Once the body vibration has dropped your vibrational level will be the same as the IDE's, allowing it to get into the body. A negative entity is an esoteric field of low vibration and depending where it sits, it can effect various organs of the body. Anunnaki and draconians normally attach in the lower abdomen and tap into the lower back through the spinal column, sending negative thoughts and attacking discs L4, L5, and L6. Over a period of time these discs become herniated. These entities also hold onto your shoulder and cause the shoulder muscles to become very tight. They drop the vibration of organs within the abdomen, like the womb, liver, pancreas, and lower intestines, causing dysfunction in these areas, and leading to sickness. It is important to remove these entities before revibrating the body. Otherwise, their presence will block meridian flow in these areas. There are also first and second dimensional entities that can lodge themselves in the hip or the shoulder or behind the eyes, which cause blockages in those areas, manifesting into various conditions like arthritis, muscle pain, and bone spurs. If you don't re-establish energy flow to the bones they start to grow incorrectly.

To remove these entities I physically grab them, pull them out and send them back to God through a portal, with Unconditional Love and forgiveness. It is not for us to judge their intent. Always let God take care of it.

Chakra Clearing

Two of the most prominent chakras that become blocked are the heart and root chakras. When any chakras are blocked, I put an esoteric pipe through that point, place an esoteric bag around the area, for instance the heart, and physically suck out and blow out the negative energy surrounding that point. When I blow out, I can physically see the low vibration that is emitted. When I can no longer see the vibration it means the chakra point is clear. Once clear, it is important to send positive energy back through the portal to revibrate the chakra and rebalance it.

Esoteric Operations

Esoteric operations are similar to regular surgery in the third dimensional world, except that the entities performing the operation are in a different dimension, and don't pierce the skin to enter the body.

If you think about it, an angelic being can't get into a low vibrational body. To perform an esoteric operation you need to raise the person's vibration to be in synch with the vibration of the angelic being. This will allow them to be able to enter the body with esoteric body parts. Esoteric body parts are created form the God Realm with the same genetic structure as your physical body parts, except that in this case, your body parts are an energy field. The angels bring in the esoteric body part, place it over the current part, and then, over a period of time, the esoteric part transposes into this dimension and your actual body part leaves this dimension and becomes esoteric. Thus, a swap has occurred. It is very important during this process to ensure that no negative entities get within the body and destroy the manifestation. That's why we say a protection prayer beforehand.

Prayer of Protection

I am of God

I ground myself to the Earth

I command you, God,

to place a bubble of 5th Dimensional,

Unconditional Love around me

to protect me from negative entities &

any fractals thereof, Manipulations

and any Transmissional Frequencies

that are not for my highest good,

*through all space/time continuum
in every dimension*

I thank You, God,

and send you my Unconditional Love

*So Be It
Amen*

This prayer must to be said every two waking hours, because the dark side evolves within two hours. If you don't, you're not protected from the dark side. The prayer is a commitment to the healing and to God to allow the manifestation to complete. You may expect a full healing, but you need to commit and exchange like energy back to God.

Breaking Soul Ties

If you have people in your life that you fell in love with, had sex with, or got close to, then you leave a part, or fractal, of your soul with that person and an energy link is formed between that fractal of your soul and their soul. When healing, it's important to break all soul ties that aren't for your highest good, cleanse them, and return all the fractals of your soul back to your body. Doing this makes you whole again. You'll find that instead of having an emotional issue with that person, you'll be able to release yourself of all trying emotional issues having to do with that person. This allows you to move onto new relationships and places, without an energy attachment.

Soul Tie Healing Example

My patient was a middle-aged female who, since age twelve, had been in and out of mental institutions. She was a prisoner in her home, as she could not go outside or into any public place. She had chronic fatigue, fibromyalgia, chronic depression, chronic lower back pain, and aching all over her body. The healing began with identifying what caused her situation, which was emotional issues. To remove these issues we began by breaking soul ties connecting her to people that weren't for her highest good. Her heart chakra was completely blocked, and stuffed full of emotion. To remove this, I created an esoteric pipe and placed it around her heart. I sucked out the negative vibration from her heart chakra and into my lungs. This took three of four times, as I continued to blow out the vibration until the smoke dissipated, indicating that the chakra was completely clear.

I have the gift of looking within the body and seeing inter-dimensional entities. I saw she had a draconian being sitting within her lower abdomen which was tapped into her L5 disc, and hanging onto her shoulders, causing the lower back issues, chronic depression, and tight muscles in her shoulders. We removed the entity and sent it back to God with Unconditional Love and forgiveness, sucked out the vibration from her abdomen, and physically combed her meridians to remove any of the blockages that were occurring. Combing the meridian involves going down the body with my hands.

I then I sent her inter-dimensional energy by opening a portal around her and beneath her, and sent her energy through her crown chakra.

Once the body was of high enough vibration the angelic beings came into the body and fit the inter-dimensional disc. We performed an esoteric operation on her damaged disc in the lower back, and replaced it with that from the angelic realm. Within 48 hours the inter-dimensional disk came into this vibration, and the original disc left this dimension. Now this lady has had a baby, and her life is completely turned around.

How to Practice Unconditional Faith

1. When doctors say you've got a certain amount of time to live, change that reality. It's your choice, not theirs. Instead of accepting a death sentence, repeat, "I'm excited about getting over this illness and for all I'm going to do in this life." Use this as an opportunity to uncover your divine gifts and be grateful for this chance to change your life. Despite what any "authority" tells you, you have the ability to heal yourself and to change your reality to one of complete wellness.

2. When faced with dire financial news, such as losing your job, change your mind set. Say, "I will get a new job. The last job was no good, and the next job will be a thousand times better." Look at leaving the old job as a blessing.

3. Changing your mindset applies to anything—airline journeys, governmental systems, crime—if you know that nothing can touch you, then nothing will. Repeat, "Nothing can harm me."

CHAPTER 5

The Divine Healing Modalities

Human beings are pure beings of light. In our optimal state we never get sick. We only become ill when something toxic creates an environment within us that allows illness to set in and grow.

In this optimal state humans are meant to express and experience unrestrained Unconditional Love. When depression, joylessness, anger, fear, frustration, confusion or hate creep in, it sets up a toxic environment where illness develops.

The following divine healing modalities are meant to explain the causes behind many illnesses and how we address them at their root source, and eliminate it from the body.

A word of caution: The healing modalities may serve as a beginning guide for lightworkers and potential healers. In addition to acquiring the knowledge of how to practice these modalities, however, it is essential for the healer to be in a pure, high vibrational state. Otherwise, the treatment is likely to be ineffective and can possibly make the situation worse.

Prayers For Divine Healing

During the process of healing it's important to say the protection prayer regularly, in order to keep the entities out while the body's vibration is precarious. Once the healing is complete and the body is at a new level of consciousness and vibration, no fungal infections or entities can get back into the body, and the prayers may be repeated less frequently.

Because negative entities evolve so quickly, individuals need to say the prayer every two hours during the healing process, barring sleep. In cases where people can't say the prayer themselves, a close family member or friend can say it for them. This is the same for children.

Prayer of Protection

I am of God

I ground myself to the earth

I command you, God,

to place a bubble of 5th dimensional,

Unconditional Love around me to protect me

*from negative entities & any fractals thereof,
manipulations and any transmissional
frequencies*

*through all space/time continuum
in every dimension*

that are not for my highest good

I thank You, God,

and send you my Unconditional Love

*So Be It
Amen*

DIVINE HEALING MODALITY

The procedure for all healing sessions, with the exception of Lyme (borrelia), AID's/HIV, and Morgellons Syndrome, contain the following elements.

1. Protection & Mirroring

If the healing session is being done by telephone or Skype, we begin every healing with a simple prayer to remove the luciferian spirit or and radionic frequencies from the listening device.

Prayer to Block Out Luciferian Spirits and Frequencies from Multimedia

I am of God

I ground myself to the Earth

I command you God to remove all the luciferian spirits & vibration from this multimedia through all space/time continuum in every dimension

I bring all the people involved with the manipulation, up through infinite levels and 20 billion light years away,

Before You, God,
for justice in only the way you know how.

I release them all to You, God, with

Unconditional Love and Forgiveness

I thank you, God,
and send you my Unconditional Love

So Be It
Amen

The next thing we do is bring the person's esoteric body into the room. What is then done to the esoteric body is mirrored in the individual's actual body. The healing process becomes exactly the same as if the person being healed is physically present in the room.

2. Grounding

To start the healing process we say a grounding prayer:

> I am of God
> I ground myself to the Earth
> I accept this healing for my highest good

3. Clearing

We then look for entities in any dimension, which reveal themselves as esoteric bodies in this dimension and become blockages. I am blessed to see these esoteric bodies – it is a gift that God of the Universe has granted me. We remove them by grabbing them, and physically pulling them from the body. Then we review and look for the energetic tattoos from the negative entities that have been embossed on their body. This symbology produces negative vibrations attracting negative entities because of the sacred geometric shapes. If we find these energetic tattoos, we eliminate them.

I say "we" and not "I" because a team of Melchizedek and Angelic Beings work with me throughout the healing process. In addition, the God Realm, or as I say, "the God of the Universe," is working with us as well. I have permission to work with the God of the Universe, the Melchizedek and Angelic Realms. (As discussed earlier, it is important for each individual to ascertain where he's from and obtain permission to work with the Angelic Realm of that dimension. In my case it's the Melchizedek Beings and Angelic Beings from that dimension).

Once I start healing I get assigned a team of Angelic Beings who work with us. They remain with the individual between sessions to ensure that the healing continues. Sometimes they start the work before I even begin.

4. Through the Portal

Once the inter-dimensional entities have been pulled out we open a portal to the Ultimate Dimension and release the entity(s) back through the portal to God, with Unconditional Love and forgiveness.

The portal is located in the ultimate dimension. This is the dimension I work with, and is where the Melchizedek Order resides.

5. Removing Residual Vibrations

Once the entity has been released through the portal, it generally leaves behind a residual negative vibration where the entity was located in the body.

To remove the residual vibration we put an "esoteric bag" over the area where the entity has been, with a pipe into my mouth. The esoteric bag is an inter-dimensional vessel of containment that takes the form of an energy field here. I inhale the negative vibration then blow it into the portal and send the negative vibration back to God.

When I blow the energy out it becomes a visible plume of vibrational smoke. I keep doing this until I can no longer see the vibration, and it becomes clear.

6. Revibration

Once the residual negative vibration is removed it is important to rebalance the individual by sending in Unconditional Love of God Energy to fill the void.

This is done by invoking angels from the Melchizedek realm to put their hands over the nearest chakra point to that area and to fire energy from their realm into the individual.

7. Meridian Combing & Unblocking

Once the area becomes warm and tingly we know the vibration is increased. We then clear the meridian lines by physical combing the actual or esoteric energy field of the person:

Upper Left

Starting from the crown, down the face and the back of the head.
Down the neck, across the left shoulder and down the left arm.
I cup my hands to collect the negative vibration from the meridian line. I then open my hands and blow through my hands at the same time. A plume of vibration will come out. If there is no vibration the meridians will appear clear. This whole process is repeated until the meridian line areas are completely clear.

Upper Right

Then we repeat the process on the right.
Start from the crown, down the face and the back of the head.
Down the neck across the right shoulder and down the right arm.
As we go out through the fingers I cup my hands to collect the negative vibration from the meridian line. I

then open my hands and blow through my hands at the same time. A plume of vibration will come out. If there is no vibration the meridians will appear clear. This whole process is repeated until that area of the meridian lines are completely clear.

Middle Left

We then comb front and back on the left side, down the neck, down the chest, and abdomen. We take the vibration out of the left hip. I cup my hands to collect the negative vibration from the meridian line. I then open my hands and blow through my hands at the same time. A plume of vibration will come out. If there is no vibration the meridians appear clear. This whole process is repeated until that area of the meridian lines are completely clear.

Middle Right

We then comb front and back on the right side, down the neck, down the chest, down abdomen, then take the vibration out of the hip on the right side. I cup my hands to collect the negative vibration from the meridian line. I then open my hands and blow through my hands at the same time. A plume of vibration will come out. If there is no vibration the meridians appear clear. This whole process is repeated until that area of the meridian lines are completely clear.

Lower Left

We then go from the hip on the left, down the side, over the knee, down the calf, then cupping my hands as it comes out of the toes. I cup my hands to collect the negative vibration from the meridian line. I then open my hands and blow through my hands at the same time. A plume of vibration will come out. If there is no vibration the meridians appear clear. This whole process is repeated until that area of the meridian lines are completely clear.

Lower Right

We then go from the hip on the right, down the side, over the knee, down the calf, then cupping my hands as comes out of the toes. I cup my hands to collect the negative vibration from the meridian line. I then open my hands and blow through my hands at the same time. A plume of vibration will come out. If there is no vibration the meridians appear clear. This whole process is repeated until that area of the meridian lines are completely clear.

8. Breaking Soul Ties and Clearing Energy Connections in this Lifetime

We ask permission from the individual to break soul ties. We grab all soul ties as directed by God, that are not for the highest good of the individual, and we bring the fractals of the soul back that were left in other people's bodies, cleanse them, and return them to the individual's body.

Steps 1-8 are performed for all healing sessions and are the same for each.

Clearing Past-Life Esoteric Transference

Esoteric transference of past life trauma can accidentally be transferred through the thin veil of this lifetime and interfere with the meridian structure. If you've been stabbed with a knife the energy field is still there, so the energy field of the implement can accidentally transfer in this lifetime. A limb chopped off, for example, might cause meridian dysfunction where there is no energy flow in that area. This traumatic situation of a past life is corrected by removing the esoteric energy field of the implement or trauma, and removing its vibrational energy.

Meridian Reactivation

After the meridians are unblocked and they are running freely, I put my right arm out just above the crown of the actual or esoteric body. I grow a vertical wall of energy below my arm, which I then sweep down the whole body from the crown to the toes.

I ask the Angelic Realm how many times this should be done, as it varies depending upon how blocked the meridians were, and complete the required number of times.

Once the meridian reactivation is complete the individual should feel a lot lighter and more clear. After several times of taking the wall of energy down, he or she should start feeling a wave of energy travelling down the body. This may take several sweeps. Normally, the quantity of sweeps varies between 15 and 23 times.

Revibration of the Body

I next open a portal from the ultimate dimension, put it around the person and close the portal beneath them so they are completely encompassed by this ultra-dimensional portal.

It's worth noting that you can lose the feeling of time when this transpires, as there is no time inside a portal.

I then invoke the angelic Melchizedek Realms from the ultimate dimension to fire energy from the individual's crown, travelling down the entire body. We know the energy is getting to the right place when the person feels tingling in his fingers and toes. It may take a few minutes for the energy to get there, depending upon how blocked the meridians were.

Once the energy is felt in the fingers and toes, we accelerate the energy by several million times, until the person either feels "floaty," or so relaxed that he feels like he is going to fall right through the bed. The sensation of feeling floaty is due to the large differential between the energy vibration, and the body vibration.

As this process is repeated during the healing sessions, the person becomes more grounded as the body vibration naturally increases.

This Healing Modality is used for every condition except for AIDS/HIV, Lyme (Borrelia) and Morgellons disease. As people with these illnesses can become too sick from the die-off as the high vibration kills off low vibration stealth pathogens and material, we instead use the Time-Space Continuum Modality.

Time-Space Continuum Modality

1. Tachyon Energy to change molecular structure

We start the treatments by using steps 1 to 7, and open a portal. Then we fire high doses of tachyon energy at the body, which rapidly reduces the percentage of the toxic substance (whether Nano-tech or pathogens) each time it's done, allowing the individual to experience no die-off symptoms.

As we near a 60% toxin reduction, we find that the toxins and co-infections begin to come back. This is caused by the toxic substances blocking the body meridians. Once the toxins have been reduced, then normal energy flow begins and the body will kill off the toxins by itself. To combat co-infections of the normal die-off, it's important to keep removing the toxins from the body on a daily basis. This step essentially changes the molecular structure of the pathogens and Nano-tech, making them benign to the body without creating die-off co-infections or toxins.

2. Tachyon Energy and the Containment Method

Morgellons and Lyme Disease have been created from primitive DNA. When this material takes hold in the body it creates a duality of space and time placing the body in two times and spaces at once. Therefore, we use tachyon energy to *tachyonize* the body and lock it back into the space-time continuum of this time.

We do this by firing tachyon energy at the body and invoking a space time continuum change, then locking it into this space and time. Thus the areas of the body effected by the primitive pathogens, which are of a past space and time, return to this space and time. The primitive DNA material cannot live in this current space and time and thus discharges from the body.

After each session, we use a containment methodology to enclose the borellia and prevent die-off, so the patient will experience little to no detrimental effect due to the toxin die-off. The containment method is similar to sending millions of jelly jars into the body, putting the toxins into the jars, then locking them in so they don't affect the body.

3. DNA Manifestation Technique

Once the toxins are 100% removed, we undertake a complete DNA manifestation to correct the DNA and make the body robust enough to inhibit future growth of the pathogens or Nano-technology.

4. Tachyon Energy to Change the Timeline

Say you've been in a car crash, and you've got a damaged leg, we tachyonize the leg and regress it back to a different timeline before the leg was traumatized, then bring it forward on a new timeline which doesn't include the trauma. This is the same energy as locking the space time continuum to the current time, used in a different way.

Esoteric Operations

Every case is different. Esoteric operations are used where something is defective, disc or spinal injuries, for example, fibroids or tumors, when new body parts are required, for diseased organs or blockages in the arteries, or when we need to break down crystallization or calcification. We use esoteric operations to correct endocrine glands and the adrenals, or when we need to build up muscles in the heart or leg, for example. We paste "celestial goo," which is a thick energy that converts to the energy it's pasted on. If a leg muscle has been paralyzed for twenty years and has atrophied, for example, the goo will build the muscle up.

Essentially, esoteric operations involve heightening the body's vibration until it reaches the same level of the Angelic Realm, enabling the Angelic Beings to enter the body and make corrections. The Beings switch slightly into this dimension and once they are inside the body, can correct the defective organ or tissues and repair anything that needs work.

Letting Go

Have absolutely no fear of anything at all, and know that God protects you.

CHAPTER 6

ILLNESSES A TO Z

The following summaries are meant to offer some understanding of the condition or disease, as well as the healing procedure used to treat it.

ADD/ADHD (also see Autism)

Individuals labeled as ADD or ADHD are normally very spiritually gifted, and therefore become bored with the 3D teaching found in school classrooms or corporate environments. The doctor's answer to ADD is to medicate, which dumbs down the spirituality and drops the vibration of the body, thus suppressing the child or adult's spiritual growth. What these individuals need is a different way of teaching and working. If a parent came to me with a child diagnosed with ADD, I would ask him to look at the child's gifts and help the child grow spiritually instead of suppressing his natural inclinations. Giving the child or adult a better understanding of why they are here, I would work on their heart chakra to give them inner peace and to raise their vibration.

Anemia

Can be caused by many things. Anemia normally arises from issues with the GI tract, causing lack of iron absorption. This can be healed by clearing the body of entities, healing emotional issues, and rebalancing. Blood Disorders can also be caused by genetics. If this is the case we implement steps 1 to 7 of the Divine Healing Modality and clear the body. Then we invoke a DNA change which will correct the defect of the genetic strands.

DNA manifestation exchanges can take place over the course of six weeks once the vibration of the body is high enough. When the DNA manifestation is complete and the whole body is rebalanced, the anemia disappears.

Allergy, Sinusitis

This can be caused by fungal infections and low vibrational material coming from the outside world. Once the sinuses are revibrated this goes away. We follow the Divine Healing modality, combing the sinus meridians and get the angelic realm to revibrate the area. We focus Unconditional Love of God Energy just on those areas.

Alzheimer's

Caused by toxins within the brain, normally because the liver vibration is low. The direct cause is emotional issues, allowing low-vibrational inter-dimensional entities to enter the liver and cause toxin build-up in the brain. Once the entity, or entities, are removed, the body is revibrated, and the toxins are gone, it is important to manifest new brain cells using esoteric operations to restore the brain cell functionality.

Aorta Valve, Arteries, Calcification, Hardening of the Arteries
(also see Heart)

Caused by calcium deposits within the arterial system. If your body isn't processing toxins and discharging properly, calcification and deposits within the arterial system develop. This is brought about by low function of the endocrine glands, specifically the adrenals and/or parathyroid. This is caused by toxins or energy blockages created by entities, where toxins fail to filter out through the bloodstream.

To heal this, we use steps 1 to 7 of the Divine Healing Modality and clear the body. Then we perform an esoteric operation by sending the Melchizedek angelic beings in to correct and retrigger the adrenals and parathyroid. Once the parathyroid is retriggered there will be no more leeching of the calcium out of the bones. We then perform an esoteric operation and send in the angelic realm to break down the calcification within the arteries or the heart valve.

Arthritis, Bone Spurs

Caused by emotional issues then entity blockages in particular parts of the body which inhibit the energy flow down those meridian lines. This lack of energy will allow the bone to crystalize and cause calcification in the joints, or bone spurs. Once the entity is removed and the body is revibrated, an esoteric operation is performed where the inter-dimensional angelic beings break down this crystallization and discharge it through the lymphatic system. The rate of breaking this calcification down depends upon the individual's metabolism. If it is done too quickly, the calcium can build within the kidneys, causing kidney stones.

To heal this, we use steps 1 to 7 of the Divine Healing Modality and clear the body. Then we perform an esoteric operation by sending the Melchizedek angelic beings to the affected area. They break down the calcification either within the joint or the bone spur that's manifested and discharge it back through the lymphatic system. This can take several sessions to clear and will not come back because there will be normal energy flow throughout the body.

Without proper energy flow crystallization takes place within joints causing arthritis or unusual growth spurs to occur within the joints and bone structure.

Autism

Due to the fact that the individual is very gifted and is in fact a Starseed, the child doesn't sit well in this 3D world because their whole genetic structure was created for the 5th dimension. When humanity evolves to the 5th dimension these individuals will fit right in. These children are generally extremely gifted, and can see inter-dimensional beings and communicate with them. They're normally unconditionally loving, but their frustration level is high because they are trapped in a body that can't properly express emotion. We could perform a DNA change in order to allow them to function correctly in this 3D world, however, it is my belief that they should be left alone and allowed to transcend as the fifth dimensional shift arises. This vibration is too low for them, now. This also applies to the ADD/ADHD children as well. The ADD/ADHD adults have for the most part learned to manage this 3D world.

Autism can also be caused by genetic defect. If this is the case, which we discover divinely, we implement steps 1 to 7 of the Divine Healing Modality and clear the body. Then we invoke a DNA change which will correct the defect of the genetic strands once the vibration is high enough. This manifestation can take between four to six weeks and will render the person "bipolar" with their emotions shifting to extremes. This is due to the fact that their DNA is changing throughout their body. It is important to repeat the prayers faithfully every two hours during this time in order to keep clearing the body.

Blood Disorders, Viral (such as Malaria) or Genetic (such as clotting disorders like Thrombosis or Hemophilia)

We implement steps 1 to 7 of the Divine Healing Modality and clear the body. Then we invoke a DNA change which will correct the defect of the genetic strands once the vibration is high enough. This manifestation can take between four and six weeks. It's important to keep the body vibration high during this time to allow the manifestation to complete. We do this with repeat sessions where we heighten the body's vibration using inter-dimensional energy and by constantly clearing the body using steps 1-7.

Brain Aneurisms, Strokes

Strokes can be caused by weak capillaries in the brain. Once the body is cleared of entities and the emotional issues are healed, an esoteric operation is performed where the angelic beings repair the damaged capillaries. The second cause can be due to 4th dimensional Draconian entities. These can enter the body and create stroke symptoms without causing any issue with the brain. Once the entity is removed, the emotional issues healed, and the body vibration is increased, the stroke symptoms completely disappear. We have seen this on many occasions.

Breast Cancer

Arises when emotional issues cause the body's vibration to drop allowing a second dimensional entity, normally a snake being, to enter and curl up within the breast. There, it blocks the complete meridian structure, because the breast then becomes low vibrational. Fungal infections can manifest within the breast, causing cysts, which turn into cancer growths. We implement steps 1 to 7 of the Divine Healing Modality and clear the body. Then we remove all the negativity from the heart chakra, remove the entity from the breast, comb the meridian structure over the breast, then revibrate the area. We then fire tachyon energy at the breast to change the molecular structure of the tumor, rendering it benign. We follow this with an esoteric operation where the angelic beings break down the tumor and discharge it through the lymphatic system. Over a period of time the tumor will shrink and disappear.

Cancer, all forms, including Brain, Liver and all forms of Lymphoma (also see Leukemia)

Cancer primarily begins with emotional disorder. The body vibration drops permitting one or more negative entities to enter, further dropping the vibration of the part of the body they are inhabiting, and allowing fungal infections to manifest. Once fungal infections arise, they generally turn into cancer growths over a period of time.

To eradicate cancer it is important to attain an understanding of what traumas have occurred to suppress the natural vibration of the body. Trauma may not always be apparent, and could have even occurred in the womb. The trauma is addressed by revisiting and releasing all emotional issues during this lifetime. Then the entity is removed and the whole body is raised to a high vibrational state. What we normally do with cancer tumors is to tachyonize them, which changes the molecular structure of the tumor and renders it benign. We then do two things. One, perform an esoteric operation allowing the angelic beings to go in and break down the tumor and discharge it through the lymphatic system. At the same time we switch the tumor out into a different space time dimension through the inter-dimensional portal. These two techniques help to rapidly reduce the tumor. It is important to get the body's vibrational state into the Godspace where the tumor will not return, as it will then be in too high a vibration.

Cancer can also be caused by toxins which drop the vibration of the body and lower the emotions. If cancer is toxin-related we normally switch it out in the space time continuum, and revibrate the liver to allow the liver to perform its normal toxin-eradication elimination process. It's very important for the individual to change eating habits, and to eat only high-vibrational, organic food that is revibrated using the food prayer.

Candida, Thrush

These are fungal infections and therefore are caused by low vibration of the body, or the mother's body at birth. We implement steps 1 to 7 of the Divine Healing Modality and clear the body. It's important to heal the emotional issues, clear the body of entities and blockages, and then fire tachyon energy to kill off the fungal infection. The angelic beings are sent in to comb out the infection that has been rendered benign, and to clear the body.

Diabetes, Hypoglycemia

If your pancreas functions perfectly, you can eat twenty cakes and your body would digest the sugar. It is important to eliminate the dogma that diabetes is caused by eating too much sugar. It is actually caused by emotional issues, which drop the vibration of the body, allowing fourth dimensional entities to enter the body and sit over the pancreas. This drops the pancreas' vibration and paralyzes it, preventing it from processing sugar properly. To eradicate this, we heal the emotional issues, after implementing steps 1 to 7 of the Divine Healing Modality and clear the body. We remove the entity, increase the general vibration of the body, and revibrate the pancreas, taking its functionality back to 100%. It's amazing that once this is complete, the blood sugar is rebalanced to the normal state.

Emotional Conditions, including Bipolar, Manic depression, Personality Disorders

Also, Healing of Ego and Self Pity, Blockages of Emotion, Drug Abuse and Alcohol Addictions, Stress Disorder, Body Issues, Distorted Body Perception, Body Paranoia, Trauma, PTS, Sexual Trauma, Rape and Sexual Abuse, Childhood Abuse, including Neglect , OCD (Childhood), Smoking, Emotional Trauma From Death, Stuttering, Domestic Violence, Violent Tendencies, Anger, and Divorce

When people come to me for healing I always ask the angelic realm to show me what emotional issues have caused the symptoms. The angelic realm plays me a video of those events in their lives to provide an understanding of why the individual is in the current space. It is then important to break ties with the assailant or cause of the abuse and bring the responsible party (s) before God and allow the client to transfer all of his emotion over to God. In my experience there is always an assailant of some kind, whether it's in human form or inter-dimensional. An assailant is not always deliberately malicious, although they often are.

We bring the assailant before God, and say the following prayer:

Emotional Release Prayer

I am of God

I ground myself to the earth

Dear God, I bring (assailant's name) before you

for Justice in only the way you know how.

through all space/time continuum

in every dimension

I realize it's not for me to judge (assailant)

Therefore I release (assailant) to you, God

with Unconditional Love and Forgiveness

I thank You, God,

and send you my Unconditional Love

So Be It
Amen

Saying this prayer with authority releases the negative energy from the heart chakra into the universe and allows God to take care of it. Therefore it becomes not your responsibility to hold onto that negativity. Once this has been done we insert an esoteric pipe through the breastbone and form an esoteric bag around the heart thus encapsulating the entire heart chakra. I physically suck out the negative vibration into my lungs, and blow it out into the universe. We then clear the body of negative entities. Once this is done several times the heart chakra becomes clear. Then Unconditional Love and God vibration is sent to the heart chakra giving the client Absolute Peace. Very often the person will get an overwhelming emotional release, either right away or in the near future. We then comb the meridian lines, activate the meridian lines, open a portal and send high vibrational love of God energy down the entire body.

It sometimes takes several sessions to completely release and get the client into a high vibrational state. By doing this all the symptoms caused by the emotional issues fade away.

Eye Issues, including Cataracts, Macular Degeneration, Blindness, Myopia and TON

We need to identify whether the issue is genetic or caused by lack of energy flow by asking divinely.

If it's genetic, such as glaucoma and macular degeneration, we implement steps 1 to 7 of the Divine Healing Modality and clear the body. Then we invoke a DNA change which will correct the defect of the genetic strands once the vibration is high enough. Once the body has reached a high vibrational state, we send in the angelic beings to perform an esoteric operation of the eye.

If someone has had trauma to the eye due to an accident, we tachyonize the eye, change the space time continuum, and take it back to a time when the eye was healthy, and then bring it back on the new timeline without the trauma. There is always a time delay between doing this and when the manifestation is complete, which can take several days. During this time it is important to keep your vibration up and not let any external vibrations or entities effect your body.

The third type is caused by physical wear, such as near-sightedness or far-sightedness, or caused by meridian blockages such as cataracts, or optic nerve trauma such as traumatic optic neuropathy or TON. We perform an esoteric operation and correct the defect by sending in the inter-dimensional Melchizedek beings once the energy blockage is removed, and after performing steps 1-7 of the Divine Healing Modality. This returns the individual to normal sight usually after seven or eight sessions, depending upon the metabolism of the individual. While we've had success bringing back 20/20 vision, it is important to maintain the correction by breaking up computer work, for instance, by looking into the distance on a regular basis.

Fibromyalgia

Fibromyalgia is a catch-all term signifying that an individual exhibits nine out of twenty-one symptoms that include depression, lower back issues, body aches, GI tract problems, tight shoulder muscles, and so on. Fibromyalgia is generally brought about by emotional issues causing the body vibration to drop and thus allowing an anunnaki or draconian inter-dimensional entity, or IDE, to enter.

To treat this, we implement steps 1 to 7 of the Divine Healing Modality and clear the body. We then focus on particular symptoms, for example the adrenals, and perform an esoteric operation to get them functioning properly. Adrenal dysfunction can cause chronic fatigue, while low liver function can cause toxic build-up in cells acting as a depository for toxins. If lower back issues are present, or if the disk has been damaged, an esoteric operation is performed to replace the disk. After the entity is removed and the symptoms addressed and rebalanced, fibromyalgia disappears.

Gall Bladder

The gall bladder normally becomes paralyzed by IDE's preventing it from working properly. These negative entities enter after an emotional issue in the person's life caused their vibration to drop. Therefore, to heal, it is important to understand and heal the emotional issue as described in the Emotional Conditions section. Once this is accomplished we remove the entity that sits over the gall bladder, comb the meridian lines, send high vibration down the entire body, then perform an esoteric operation where the angelic realm puts their hands around the gall bladder to revibrate it. Then Melchizedek beings go in and comb the meridian structure of the gall bladder, breaking down the hard bile deposits that cause gall stones and allowing them to flush out through the lymphatic system. It can take several sessions to break down the bile deposits and to trigger the gall bladder's full function, which occurs in stages. Sadly, the medical solution to gall bladder issues is to cut the organ out. God intended for us to have a gall bladder and thus created it. It's major function is to aid digestion of fat and without one the individual will almost always suffer from digestive issues.

Genetic "defects" causing Cystic Fibrosis, Huntington's, Parkinson's, Muscular Dystrophy, Rheumatoid Arthritis, Creutzfeldt-Jakob Disease, Downs syndrome, Epilepsy, Hodgkin's Disease, and Spinal Bifida

Genetic defects can come about for a variety of reasons. It is important to get the individual's body vibration to the highest Godspace of Unconditional Love and Inner Peace by removing all negative entities, removing all emotional issues, opening a portal and sending Unconditional Love of God energy down the individual's body until they get to that space. A DNA change can not take place without the body being in a high vibrational space. Once the body has achieved this state a DNA manifestation begins, which starts at the sacrum point and manifests outwards throughout the entire body. The DNA change takes between 4-6 weeks, allowing time for every cell in the body to be altered. It is vital for the individual being healed to completely protect himself during this time. If anything negative gets back into the body the DNA manifestation will be shut down. The individual must commit, and repeat the Prayer of Protection every two hours while awake for the duration of the healing. Once the DNA manifestation is complete the symptoms and illness will subside.

GI, Wheat Intolerance, Food Intolerance, Colon, Stomach, Intestinal Issues, IBS, Crohns, Reflux, Celiac

From experience, I've found that most gastrointestinal issues are caused by negative blockages within the GI tract. These blockages are caused by IDE's which have entered the body due to a lowered vibration, generally having dropped because of emotional trauma, or infection by toxins. Unless these entities are removed they will paralyze the intestines or body part where they are sitting.

When healing the intestinal and stomach area we remove the blockages, address the trauma that caused the issue, then heal the damage to the intestinal structure creating the symptoms, whether they be acid reflux, bowel obstructions, or a digestive imbalance that is creating holes in the intestinal lining. Holes are healed, for instance, by sending in the Angelic and Melchizedek Beings to perform an esoteric operation and rebalance the areas, and reconstructing the intestinal lining so that the holes diminish. Then we revibrate the gastrointestinal tract and raise the vibration of the entire intestinal structure so the food goes down at the same rate and is absorbed in the correct part of the intestines. If you can imagine the situation where if the lower intestine is paralyzed, the food goes down at a normal rate until it reaches the paralyzed area, then begins backing up. It is therefore digesting in the wrong area of the intestine, causing acid reflux and burning, and also depriving the body of nutrition. These holes can affect the absorption rate of things like wheat and foods containing gluten, causing inflammation where the holes are located. This is called leaky gut syndrome, and it can cause someone to be underweight because they're not absorbing the proper nutrients although they're eating a normal amount of food.

No matter what the gastric issue is, it's important to use the Food Prayer before meals in order to remove anything from the food that is not of God, such as genetic modifications (GMO's), to optimize the food's nutritional value, and to rebalance the karma associated with eating animal products. If an animal has had a difficult life or experienced fright or pain when it was slaughtered, that vibration of suffering, fright and pain is imprinted on the meat. It's important to rebalance and increase the vibration of the food so it doesn't effect your spirituality.

Food Prayer

Put your hands around the plate while looking at the food, and say with complete authority, so that you feel a spiritual "shiver" indicating that the prayer is working:

I am of God

I ground myself to the Earth

I command you, God, to correct & rebalance any modifications made to this food that are not of God

through all space/time continuum
in every dimension

optimize the nutritional value of this food, remove all its toxins

and bless the souls of the animals and plants that have given their life
to provide nutrition to my body

I thank you, God,

and send you my Unconditional Love

So Be It
Amen

This prayer should be said before all meals, and before anything that is eaten or drunk.

Hearing Loss (genetic or blocked canals, or due to nerve damage)

Hearing Loss can be caused by a number of things, normally low vibration of the ear, or a defect within the inner ear. We implement steps 1 to 7 of the Divine Healing Modality and clear the body. As in the previous section, we clear emotional issues, comb the meridians, revibrate the body, then once the body vibration is high enough, the Angelic and Melchizedek Beings come in and perform an esoteric operation within the inner ear.

Bacterial and Viral Infections, including Meningitis, Herpes, Epstein Barr, Mononucleosis

We implement steps 1 to 7 of the Divine Healing Modality and clear the body.
We comb the meridian lines and revibrate the body to a point of Unconditional Love and get it into the Godspace. We then send tachyon energy into the body, using space-time continuum energy to change the molecular structure of the bacterial or viral infection. Thus turning it into something benign to the body. This kills the infection and the benign material is discharged through the lymphatic system. Keeping the body in a high vibrational Godspace will ensure that the infection doesn't return, as no infection can live in a high vibrational body.

Heart Issues, MVP, Mitochondrial Disease, Pulmonary Edema

There are a few causes of heart issues. If an IDE is sitting over the heart causing a low vibrational blockage, it can suppress the heart and paralyze the muscles, keeping it from normal functionality and bringing about atrial fibrillation and blood disorders. There can also be deposits on the valves caused by the IDE paralyzing the parathyroid, which leaches calcium from the bones. If the adrenals are dysfunctional and not filtering out the deposits, the calcium will collect within the arterial lining, and the heart valves, prohibiting them from closing completely, and therefore leaving the valves stuck open. A virus of the blood can leave behind deposits and clog the valve, or create neuropathic problems where the nerves aren't triggering the heart properly because the controls are being interfered with. All these things make the muscles weak. If the valves aren't closed, the heart is working harder and can cause enlargement of the heart.

First we implement steps 1 to 7 of the Divine Healing Modality and clear the body.

We remove the entity and revibrate the heart. If the muscles are weak we take celestial goo and recreate the muscle tissue. When this thick celestial goo energy comes in contact with the muscle it recreates this muscle with the same DNA of the body, thus rebuilding the heart muscle. If there are deposits on the valve it's important to undergo an esoteric operation. Once the energy is high enough the Angelic and Melchizedek Beings go in and break down the deposits on the heart valves so as to discharge the material through the lymphatic system. This can take several sessions.

Hormonal Disorders (male and female), Menopause, PMS, Post Partum Depression

We implement steps 1 to 7 of the Divine Healing Modality and clear the body.

Hormonal disorders are dealt with by combing the meridian lines and revibrating the body to a point where the body never gets sick. We then send the Angelic Beings in and they rebalance the hormone glands and revibrate the area by placing their hands over the endocrine areas, including the pituitary gland, pancreas, ovaries, testes, thyroid gland, and adrenal glands, and fire energy into the region. We then send in the Melchizedek Beings to perform an esoteric operation, to comb these glands out and rebalance them so they all work in synch with one another. Thus rebalancing the whole body's hormonal system. This may take a few sessions to complete.

Inter-dimensional Implants

Inter-dimensional implants are generally the result of abduction by the zeta greys, who use technological instruments to shut down the pineal gland and monitor the body. We use tachyon energy, which is in the form of electrostatic energy, to fry the implant and make it inoperable, thus rendering it benign to the body. We then send in the Angelic Beings to break down the residue and discharge it through the lymphatic system.

Kidney and Adrenal Issues

Kidney and Adrenal Issues can be caused by stress, leading to IDE's within the abdomen. We implement steps 1 to 7 of the Divine Healing Modality and clear the body. We remove the entity, comb the meridian structure, heighten the vibration of the body and the kidneys individually, then send in the Angelic Beings to balance the adrenal glands and restart them. This will increase the body's energy because adrenal dysfunction causes chronic fatigue. It is important to keep the body in a high vibrational state where the entities cannot get back in.

Leukemia, Liver Disorders, Lupus, Gout, Cirrhosis

The liver can be blocked by toxins or low vibrations, where the IDE has gotten into the abdomen and is sitting over the liver. Toxins can paralyze the liver with their overwhelmingly low vibration. If the liver drops below 20% then leukemia results, because the toxins aren't being filtered from the body and are destroying the platelets.

The symptoms always start off by emotional issues or toxins. We implement steps 1 to 7 of the Divine Healing Modality and clear the body. We comb the meridian lines, activate the meridian lines, open a portal and send high vibrational Love Of God Energy down the entire body. The portal is opened and the toxins are switched out through the space and time continuum to a different dimension. In doing this the client experiences either a drawing sensation away from the body or a cool breeze leaving the body.

For leukemia, we revibrate the liver locally, where the Angelic Beings place their hands around the liver and revibrate it to 100% functionality. The liver doesn't maintain its vibration the first time, so it's generally necessary to revibrate several times in order to maintain normal liver function, which is generally between 90-100% vibration, depending upon its function. Once the liver has attained 90-100% functionality depending upon what the liver is processing, whether it be foods, alcohol or other liquid. Once the body vibration is high enough, we can then get the Angelic Beings to recreate the platelets in the bone marrow. After several sessions the platelet count will drastically increase and the white blood cell count will be rebalanced.

With cirrhosis, it's important to remove the emotion that has likely caused the individual's need for escapism through alcohol or drugs. This 3D world is difficult to live in unless you are identifying your blessings and living in the Godspace. We remove and break all soul ties and remove the memory and vibration as well as the negative emotional imprint from the heart chakra. Doing this takes away the need to use substances, and provides an inner peace. Once the need for substances is removed, we do an esoteric operation on the liver and replace it with an esoteric liver. Within several days the third dimensional liver is replaced by the energy field liver as they switch dimensions. The third dimensional liver disappears and the esoteric one becomes the actual liver. It's important during this time to keep the body vibration to a very high rate as the esoteric liver energy field will get squashed, and the manifestation will be cancelled, if any negativity gets back in.

Liver disorders can also be caused by Lyme disease, so it is important to check for borrelia stealth pathogens, which completely block the meridian structure of the liver (please see section on Lyme). Lupus is caused by the toxin die-off of borrelia (see Lyme section). Gout is caused by excess uric acid in the system not being filtered by the liver.

Loss of Spirituality, Low Spiritual Awareness

Spiritual awareness can be suppressed by a number of factors. First is fluoride, which crystalizes the pineal gland and suppresses the function of the spiritual third eye and the ability to see auras, energy fields and a whole lot more. This spiritual eye is your direct connection to God. When your spiritual eye is not working you're functioning in the low vibration of the third dimensional world where your emotions are suppressed to the point that you don't feel joy or anything but numbness. Numbness is the state where nothing really matters. When someone dies you feel melancholy, which is the expression of emotion over the loss. When the third eye is shut down you don't express emotion at all.

The second cause is generally an IDE blockage that is dropping the vibration of the body, causing depression by tapping into the lower back, and sending negative thoughts that hinder your spiritual awareness. Pineal and pituitary function goes hand in hand with a high vibrational body. When your vibration is low it affects these glands, causing your spiritual vibration to be radically reduced.

To heal this we implement steps 1 to 7 of the Divine Healing Modality and clear the body. We get the Melchizedek beings to put their hands over the third eye and fire energy into the pineal and pituitary glands to revibrate them. Once this energy has been achieved we ask the Angelic Beings to come in and break down the crystal structure that has formed around the pineal and pituitary, thus completely reopening the third eye.

You can tell when your third eye is completely open, because when you walk outside you will see the world as if through a high definition TV. When you look at a tree you will see the definition of every leaf and every color of every leaf with clarity. Everything becomes crystal clear, including auras.

Lung Defects, Chronic Bronchitis, Emphysema, Tuberculosis

Lung issues are caused by fungal infections, contaminants of low vibration infiltrating the lungs.

We implement steps 1 to 7 of the Divine Healing Modality and clear the body. We send energy down to clear the heart chakra, detach all the soul ties and then the individual is ready to be healed. We then fire energy into the lungs, and if the lungs have an infection we tachyonize the contaminant and change its molecular structure to something benign for the body. We send in the Melchizedek Beings to comb out the contaminant. Tachyon energy is used to remove the contaminant or infection, then we revibrate the lungs and bronchial tract by firing energy through the heart and navel chakras so that the Angelic Beings can come in and comb out any residual benign contaminants.

Once the lungs are of high vibration nothing can affect them. You'll no longer get infections, for they can't live in a high vibrational body.

Lyme Disease, the stealth pathogen Borrelia, AIDS /HIV

All stealth pathogens are manmade, produced in a virus lab and released. There are many that have been geo-engineered at Fort Dietrich, and released through terraforming and chemtrails the world over.

Borrelia, which is called Lyme disease, is a stealth pathogen. This means it changes paths very quickly, and the autoimmune system must spend all of its energy hunting it down, yet is never finds it because the pathogen keeps morphing into something else. If the condition is not treated the autoimmune system crashes and allows cancer or some other opportunistic disease to come in and consume the body, when the body most lacks the ability to fight it. We have seen that the only effective treatment is to tachyonize the pathogens and co-infections, which changes their molecular structure to something benign to the body. The beauty of tachyonizing borrelia is that there are no die-off symptoms. Remember, no disease can manifest in a high vibrational body. If you send Reiki or even high dimensional God energy in, the individual might become even sicker or go into analeptic shock. It's important as a healer not to send normal energy into the body when dealing with Lyme as well as AIDS. The co-infections and toxins from borrelia are ammonia, bartonella, babecia, bbtox, Epstein-Barr, and herpes.

We start the treatments by performing steps 1 through 7 of the Divine Healing Modality, clearing the meridian lines, opening a portal, and firing high dosages of tachyon energy to rapidly but incrementally reduce the percentage of borrelia with no die off symptoms. As we near a 60% borrelia reduction, we find that the toxins and co-infections begin to come back. This is because borrelia blocks the meridians of the body. Once the borrelia has been reduced by 60% normal energy flow returns, enabling your body to kill off the borrelia by itself. To combat the co-infections of the normal die-off once we get to this level, it's important to keep removing the toxins from your body on a daily basis. Once the borrelia is 100% removed, it is time to do a complete DNA manifestation to correct the DNA and make it robust enough to repel borrelia in the future.

After each session we use the containment methodology to lock away any remaining pathogens so that die-off doesn't affect the body.

Antibiotics will help the co-infections but not the borrelia itself. These drugs present the appearance of killing the Lyme by alleviating the symptoms but not killing the borrelia, which replicates in the body extremely quickly, until reaching end stage Lyme where the immune system crashes. I have had many clients at end stage Lyme who are now back to normal.

It's important to space the healing sessions no more than four days apart to prevent the borrelia from coming back, and to stay ahead of the replication process. The key is to kill off more than is replicated. The whole process can take up to four to six months, depending upon how long its been in the body and how much it's replicated. Each individual is different.

The technique is exactly the same for AIDS. Like Lyme, HIV replicates in the body and crashes the immune system. Both pathogens are similar and the treatment for AIDS/HIV is the same as it is for Lyme.

Morgellons Syndrome

Morgellons was first invented in the 1930's during the Nazi era. The Nazis were given the technology by the Zeta greys, an alien race that traded technology in exchange for the freedom to perform abductions to experiment on the human race. It seems that the DNA material for Morgellons came from "black goo" dating back millions of years and which came from drilling into the center of the earth. Black goo doesn't have the suite of chakra points that humans currently possess, and among others, is missing the heart chakra, which deals with love, marking this DNA as extremely primitive. This goo, combined with Nano-technology from computer chips, and with borrelia (Lyme disease) delivered through chemtrails, form a substance which replicates exponentially in the body, with alarming effects.

The DNA of this primitive substance possesses only three chakra points. Your DNA make-up determines how it replicates in your body. Elements of this goo are contained in facial fillers that get rid of wrinkles and will expose you to Morgellons, by the way. Because of the rate in which it replicates, it takes over the body, changing its space time continuum and placing the body in two worlds at once: in the now, and millions of years ago when the DNA existed.

Not only are we using tachyon energy to change the structure of this Nano-biological material, but we can tachyonize the whole body and lock it back into the space / time of the now. By doing this, the material can't live in the body. It is in the wrong space / time continuum and it leaves in droves. Thus, coming out through the skin, feces and urine.

Spiritually, the clients who have Morgellons always have an energetic tattoo of symbology embossed on their body. Therefore, it is extremely important to remove these tattoos of energy. We start the treatments by performing steps 1 through 7 of the Divine Healing Modality, clearing the meridian lines, and opening 4 portals. These work in conjunction with each other in the fifth, twelfth and the Ultimate Dimension. After that, we then place an esoteric merkaba field over the portals to bring them together so they work in conjunction with each other. To create the esoteric merkaba field, use the Merkaba Field Prayer of Protection at the end of this section.

Next, we fire a very high dosage of inter-dimensional Unconditional Love energy taking it up to a level of 680 trillion times strong. Due to the high dosage of energy, this removes any trace of the energy tattoos on their body. Once the energetic tattoos are eradicated, we reduce the Unconditional God energy down to 3.4 trillion times strong. Next we fire high dosages of Tachyon energy again at 3.4 trillion times strong to rapidly and incrementally reduce the foreign substances with no die-off symptoms. As we near a 60% reduction, we find that the toxins and co-infections begin to come back. This is because the nanotech and borrelia block the meridians of the body. As soon as these substances have been reduced, normal energy flow returns, enabling their body to kill off the borrelia by itself. To combat the co-infections of the normal die-off as we get to this level, it's important to keep removing the toxins from your body on a daily basis. When the substances are 100% removed, it is time to do a complete DNA manifestation to correct the DNA. Thus, making it robust enough to repel re-infection in the future. This Modality rapidly heals the body of Morgellons.

It's important not to have more than four days between each healing session, or the substances creating the disease will return. The key is to kill off more than is replicated. The whole process can take up to four to six months, depending upon how long it's been in your body and how much it's replicated.

Some types of Nano-technologies are activated by military frequencies sent from satellites, which create additional pain and discomfort within the body. These frequencies are 10^{12}Hz. Having this Nano-technology in your body provides outside sources with the means of monitoring your body, checking the impact of the technologies and its effect.

We then use tachyon energy to lock the time into the right now. This can take several days to complete, with the whole process spanning several months.

The Merkaba Field of Protection Prayer

I am of God

I ground myself to the Earth

I command you God to create an esoteric merkaba field around me

to protect me from any negative entities, manipulations and transmissional frequencies that are not for my highest good

Program this merkaba with the blueprint of my DNA and the Keys of Enoch so as not to allow anything to enter except for my highest good

in all space and time, in every dimension

I thank you God

and send you my Unconditional Love

So Be It
 Amen

Neuropathy, Nerve Ending Damage

Can be caused by ingesting toxins affecting the body's imbalance which affect the DNA of your body, allowing various symptoms of neuropathy to occur. To heal this we remove the toxins by opening a portal over the body and switching the toxins through the space time continuum to the ultimate dimension. Then we implement steps 1 to 7 of the Divine Healing Modality and clear the body. We revibrate the adrenals and the liver and perform an esoteric operation on the adrenals once revibrated to stimulate them to 100% functionality. Then we perform an esoteric operation with the Melchizedek Beings, who repair the damaged nerve endings.

Once the vibration of the body is high enough, we go in and repair the DNA strands as necessary by invoking a DNA change, repairing the strands that are causing the dysfunction and bringing the DNA back to the blueprint. The DNA change cannot be invoked unless the body vibration is high enough.

If the nerve damage has been caused by the co-infection and toxins of Lyme Disease die-off, please see the Lyme section.

Obesity & Weight Issues

Obesity can be caused by three things. The first is overeating, that occurs because food these days possesses twenty percent of the nutrients it did thirty years ago. An entire plate of food only provides 20% of your body's necessary nutrients, while in the past it would have provided all of them. After eating your body's craving for food causes you to eat more in order to satisfy its thirst for nutrients.

To correct this we say the Food Prayer, revibrating food back to 100% of its nutritional value. This way eating 20% of the amount of food you are used to will cause your body to become full. I've seen people lose weight very quickly using this prayer. It is important to say it each time you take a substance into your body, fully, and with conviction. Of course it's important to eat a balanced and healthy diet, for junk food can only be revibrated to a low level nutritional value.

The second way obesity can occur is through a drop in vibration of the liver. This is caused by emotional issues dropping the body's vibration, allowing fourth dimensional entities (IDE's) to get in. These IDE's sit over the liver, dropping its vibration, preventing the liver from processing the body's toxins. As a safety mechanism, the body puts the toxins in a repository of fat cells. This way people become obese without overeating. It is the body's mechanism of protection at work.

To heal this, we implement steps 1 to 7 of the Divine Healing Modality, clear the heart chakra, remove the IDE, and revibrate the liver until it's functioning at 100%. The body will then discharge the fat cells because they have no further use.

The third way obesity occurs is through comfort eating in order to feel better about yourself, or to create a blanket against stress, hurt or perceived danger. This correlates to our food containing only 20% of its true nutritional value, thus requiring that we eat far more to produce a satisfying feeling. To heal this, we address the emotional issues and remove them, then get the client to revibrate every bit of food or beverage that goes into his mouth.

Operation Problems, Tattoos, Surgery, Piercings

Invasive surgery or needles inserted into your skin break the meridian lines and alter the body's flow of energy. Sometimes this imbalance prevents the body from healing. It's important that after invasive actions of the skin, the meridians are repaired so that the energy flow is balanced and not blocked.

To reconnect the meridian lines, we use an esoteric operation where Angelic and Melchizedek beings go in and reconnect the meridians. First we perform steps 1 through 7 of the Divine Healing Modality. Once the vibration of the body is high enough the Angelic Beings are sent in to reconnect the meridian lines.

Osteoporosis

Osteoporosis is caused by incorrect functioning of the parathyroid gland. When this gland is imbalanced the body leeches calcium into the bloodstream, weakening the bones over a period of time. This process can cause other problems as well, for instance, with the adrenal glands. If your adrenals are not functioning properly and are being affected by the blockage, then the calcium is not being filtered out of the bloodstream. Because of this the calcium deposits elsewhere in the body, such as in the heart valve or arteries, which will, over a period of time cause issues with the circulatory system.

To heal this, we perform steps 1 through 7 of the Diving Healing Modality. Once the body is clear we revibrate the adrenal glands and parathyroid, and perform an esoteric operation where the Angelic Beings go in, clear and restart the adrenals and parathyroid. It can take several sessions to get both back to normal functionality. We also then look at the entire body and remote view in order to see what damage the excess calcium may have caused throughout the body, and we work on the areas where calcification build up has occurred. This might be within the aortic valve or the arteries, as calcium build-up generally occurs here.

To remove calcium build-up the Angelic Beings perform an esoteric operation to break down the calcium. Once the adrenal glands are restarted, the excess calcium filters out of the system. To strengthen the bones that have lost their calcium, the Angelic Beings use a celestial "goo," a thick energy, which they paste on the bones. When the goo touches bodily material it converts into that material with the same DNA. This part of the process can take several sessions. By constantly pasting celestial goo on the bones, they build up to a normal strength.

Phantom Pain

The first cause of phantom pain is amputation. When a limb is amputated the meridian structure remains in place despite the physical limb having been removed. Because of this, pain can still be felt through the meridian structure.

To remove phantom pain we perform steps 1 through 7 of the Divine Healing Modality. We then sever the meridian structure to the point where the limb has been removed and reform it around the stump of the area. In this way the meridian structure is completely removed, eliminating the phantom pain.

Phantom pain can also occur through esoteric transference of past life trauma. For example, if you have been killed by a dagger through the abdomen in the past, the thin energy field of this dimension can allow the energy field of the trauma to come through as you are born. We deal with this transference by removing the esoteric energy field of the trauma. It is important to point out that transference is not karma occurring to balance some past event, because you are born with no karma in this lifetime. Esoteric transference is actually due to the veil between the 5th and third dimensions being thin enough for the transference to mistakenly slip through. The effect on the body of this energy field, is to interfere with the meridian structure. To correct this we first need to remove the esoteric energy field by pulling out the energy field of the implement or past trauma, or remove its vibrational energy. Once this is done we perform steps 1 through 7 of the Divine Healing Modality, then we work on the area to reconnect the meridian structure by sending in Angelic Beings. The phantom pain thus disappears and the body is rebalanced back to its normal meridian flow.

Prostate

Inflammation and cancer is caused by either IDE's creating blockages in the lower abdomen, or by toxins. To correct this we perform steps 1 through 7 of the Divine Healing Modality. Once the portal is open we remove all the toxins by switching the space time continuum to a different dimension. Once this is done we send the Angelic Beings into the GI tract and the prostate to break down any enlargement, infection or cancer. If cancer is present we use tachyon energy to fry the cancer cells, and change the molecular structure of the tumor into material that is benign for the body. At this point the individual will feel a muscle burning, relief type feeling in that area as the tumor's structure changes and dies off. Once the tumor is rendered benign, we break it down and discharge it through the lymphatic system.

Schizophrenia

Caused by a significant spiritual attack, where IDE's become attached to the client, and where the client tends to befriend the entity. How do we deal with this? We have to first talk to the client and open their mind to the understanding that the IDE is there to manipulate them and not there for their highest good. When the IDE is removed, and the individual becomes tranquil and is no longer hearing voices, he might miss the company of the IDE and invite it back in, unless the individual possesses a complete understanding of the manipulation.

Once the individual has this understanding of the negative entity manipulation we can then heal by performing steps 1 through 7 of the Divine Healing Modality. We then clear the anxiety of the trauma caused by these entities by placing an *esoteric bag* over the heart chakra point and sucking out all the negative vibration associated with this emotional trauma. We then fire energy into the heart chakra, giving him a sense of overwhelming peace.

The individual must be sure to say the Energy Prayer every two hours during the course of healing, in order to complete the shift from befriending the IDE, to never again inviting it back in. The healing can take several sessions because it's important to get the body to a vibration level of Christ Consciousness. When this is achieved the entities can no longer go near the client because his high vibration will be too strong.

Sexual Dysfunction

There are a few causes of sexual dysfunction. If a marriage is in trouble, anxiety can cause this dysfunction and shut off sexual desires. If you go near someone who doesn't really want you, your sexual function can disappear. If there has been trauma from abuse, the sexual function can be compromised due to lack of self worth. That's why we do counseling with whole families in order to get them integrated, balanced and closer together, functioning as a strong and dynamic unit. Then we work on each party to remove emotional blockages, helping them to achieve inner peace and comfort, both with themselves and their partner. Taking medication to increase sexual function does not address the true self esteem issues and level of comfort with yourself or your partner. If you are comfortable with your partner, your libido will increase.

To heal, we perform steps 1 through 7 of the Divine Healing Modality. We then clear out the heart chakra by sucking out trauma with the esoteric bag over the heart, and remove all negative vibration. This will move the parties into a state of peace where they can be comfortable with one other. We clear past life issues using the Past Life Clearing Prayer, removing any cellular memory or esoteric transference associated with their past lives or past life associations with one another.

Structural Issues like Skeletal Trauma

Skeletal trauma is brought about by some physical incident that has damaged the skeleton or created fractures to the bone structure. If the energy flow in the body is compromised by meridian blockage then the bones won't heal. Therefore we clear the body of energy blockages and get the body vibration to a much higher level and closer to higher consciousness. We begin by performing steps 1 through 7 of the Divine Healing Modality. We then perform an esoteric operation on the part of the body requiring healing. Once the body is of high enough vibration the Angelic Beings can go in and correct the areas that need attention through an inter-dimensional portal.

Skin Issues, Psoriasis, Cellulite, Eczema

Skin issues are generally caused by stress or toxins. It's amazing how many people are contaminated by pathogens or toxins that they don't understand. These can manifest in the body after exposure to chemical trails, genetically modified foods, pesticides on foods, or that are present in the environment in general. The existence of these pathogens or toxins is compounded if the client has an IDE blockage dropping the vibration of the adrenal glands or liver, which directly affects the body's ability to process toxic substances, and causing the toxins to collect in fat cells beneath the skin. When obese people who eat very little are quite large, it is often due to this fact. If emotional issues are present the vibration of the liver will drop preventing the body from processing toxins as it should.

To heal, we perform steps 1 through 7 of the Divine Healing Modality. We then switch out all the toxins via the space time continuum. The individual will feel a cool breeze or a drawing sensation as if something is leaving their body. We then call in the Melchizedek Order to revibrate the kidneys, adrenals and liver, creating a warm and tingly feeling. Once the kidneys are of a high enough vibration we call in the Angelic Beings to perform an esoteric operation to clear the adrenal glands causing them to start functioning properly. As the liver vibration increases and reaches 60-80 % functionality the individual experiences a great clearing in his head as toxins are processed by the liver. Once the liver function reaches 100%, and the toxins are switched by the space time continuum, the Angelic Beings comb the fat cells just beneath the skin and remove the toxins that are affecting the skin itself. Finally, we clear anxiety from the heart chakra using the esoteric bag and detach any past life connections, and break any soul ties in this lifetime. The whole procedure may take several sessions.

Sleep Disorders

Normally caused by emotional blockage or hormonal imbalance. To heal this we perform steps 1 through 7 of the Divine Healing Modality. We then use the esoteric bag to remove all anxiety. We follow this by firing high energy into the heart chakra, giving the individual an overwhelming sense of peace. We say the Past Life Clearing Prayer to make sure there is no esoteric transference.

If sleep disorders are caused by hormonal imbalance it's important to revibrate the reproductive area and the spleen, then send in the Angelic Beings to rebalance the hormonal secretion glands. Hormonal issues are generally caused by an entity blockage. Even menopause shouldn't be a bad experience. A blockage will unbalance hormones, compounding the symptoms while a normal menopause should be tranquil.

Spinal and Lower Back Issues

People are essentially built for hunting, running and athletic pursuits. So, why do so many people have spinal issues, degeneration of discs and vertebrae, when the spine is one of the most prominent elements of your body, holding your entire skeletal structure together?

There is a clear cause of skeletal issues, which is external to the body. Spines should not degenerate, and discs should not herniate or compress. Our experience has been that all spinal issues are caused by IDE energy blockages. Once an IDE gets within the lower abdomen and attaches itself, it lodges in the lower back, normally at the L4 or L5 disc, and drains the body's *merkaba* energy field, sending negative thoughts through the spinal cord. As the IDE holds on through the shoulders or head, it compresses the spine, causing scoliosis and tightening of the spinal muscles, completely blocking the meridian flow down the spine and causing the vertebra joints to calcify.

An automobile or other type of accident can also cause trauma to the spine. Trauma and pain drops the body's vibration, allowing IDE's to enter making the pain and injury far worse. Additional pain drops the body vibration further, thus compounding symptoms.

To heal these issues, we perform steps 1 through 7 of the Divine Healing Modality. We then ask the Melchizedek Beings to revibrate the spine by putting their inter-dimensional hands just below the skull and at the sacral point at the beginning of the spine, revibrating the whole area. Then we send in the Angelic Beings to perform an esoteric operation where they replace discs or vertebrae with inter-dimensional replacements. The esoteric discs come into this dimension, while the existing discs leave this dimension, thus replacing the discs of the damaged areas over the course of a few days. While this is happening it is imperative that the Prayer of Protection is repeated every two waking hours. If an IDE gets in during this time it will destroy the energy field and render the manifestation useless, and the process will need to be repeated.

Teeth

Some people are born with weak teeth. This is compounded by the fluoride added to water supplies, toothpastes, and other products, which causes our teeth to weaken instead of making them healthier. Issues with teeth can also be genetic, or can stem from infections resulting from autoimmune problems.

To heal the teeth, we perform steps 1 through 7 of the Divine Healing Modality. We then ask the Melchizedek Beings to revibrate the area by putting their hands around the jaw and firing energy into the mouth, teeth, gums, dental structure, and jaw.

We send in the Angelic Beings to perform an esoteric operation where they paste the thick and energetic *celestial goo*, to increase dental strength. If the teeth are damaged, new teeth are placed in energy fields over the current teeth, which will swap dimensions over several days, thus replacing the teeth.

If the teeth issues are caused by genetics, we get the client's energy high enough to where we can invoke a DNA exchange manifestation, which takes four to six weeks to complete. Once this manifestation takes place we find that the teeth become stronger and revert to the natural state of the DNA blueprint. A DNA manifestation must wait until the individual's vibration is high enough so that it will stick.

Bacterium and toxins can alter the state of your genetics. The DNA blueprint you came here with is radically changed by the agrobacterium coming from, among other things, GMO foods, altering your genetics.

Thyroid, Endocrine

The endocrine system consists of the thyroid, parathyroid, adrenals and spleen, all of which are affected by IDE energy blockages. Whether it's a fourth dimensional entity sitting within your abdomen, or a second dimensional being sitting over your parathyroid or throat, it will affect the functionality of your glands. The glands directly affect the body's energy level. The parathyroid also affects the body's calcium level, which is addressed further in the section on osteoporosis.

To heal this we perform steps 1 through 7 of the Divine Healing Modality. We then perform an esoteric operation on the thyroid, parathyroid, adrenals, and the spleen, where necessary, to retrigger these glands and take them to normal functionality. This can take several sessions.

Trauma from Abduction

From experience, we have found abduction trauma to be affecting many thousands of people. The abductions have taken place primarily by the zeta greys, who entered an agreement with our government representatives, allowing them to freely abduct high numbers of various human beings in exchange for technology. This came about because the zeta greys lost their ability to reproduce, causing them to experiment with human embryos and sperm in order to recreate their own race. In mid 2013 the galactic federation ordered the zeta greys to leave, so these abductions are no longer taking place. There are good abductions as well as destructive ones, wherein the abductee is educated. After the abduction they can wipe the conscious memory while leaving in place the information contained in the subconscious. Many times the zeta greys left implants in abductees in order to monitor them. These implants take many forms, and block spirituality.

To heal this, we perform steps 1 through 7 of the Divine Healing Modality. We then release all the trauma that is imbedded in the heart chakra, and bring the responsible parties before God for justice in only the way God knows how, and get the client to release them with Unconditional Love and forgiveness.

Then we remote view the body to look at where the implants are located. We fire infinite dimension tachyon energy at the implants, which changes their molecular structure into material benign to the body and rendering them inoperable. The implants are then broken down by the body's immune system and are discharged by the lymphatic system.

Viral Issues such as Hemophilia, Hepatitis, Jaundice

Viral-based diseases can stem from a variety sources, including the air or from transmission by other individuals. The way to heal is to implement steps 1 through 7 of the Divine Healing Modality, then send high levels of vibrational energy down and through the body. We remove all soul ties in this lifetime, and clear the heart chakra of emotional issues. Over several sessions the body will raise to a vibration too high for the virus to live in. For the more serious conditions like hepatitis, we use tachyon energy to change the molecular structure into something benign for the body, then kill it off. This can take several sessions to raise the body to a level of Christ Consciousness, thus preventing viral infections from living in the body.

Womb Issues, Fibroids, Endometriosis, Reproduction, Infertility, Tubal Pregnancies, Fertility

In my experience womb issues are formed by entity blockages. When the vibration of the womb drops, it stops meridian flow and sets the whole womb area off balance, including the ovaries. Fungal and yeast infections can manifest, causing endometriosis, ovarian cysts, fibroids, and uterine cancer. The IDE's entered due to emotional trauma, or through sex with a low vibrational person. If you open your base chakra up to someone, no amount of prayer can block entities from passing through to you. When a man of low vibration ejaculates into a woman, his sperm, which is also of low vibration, will drop the vibration of the woman's womb. It's important to ensure that partners are in synch with each other's energy.

As with the other issues, we implement steps 1 through 7 of the Divine Healing Modality, address the emotional trauma and release it, clear the heart trauma, remove the entity, do an esoteric operation to break down the fibroids or correct the womb lining, and comb the meridian structure of the womb so that the problem never occurs again. (For ovarian cancer, please refer to the cancer section)

It All Comes Back to Unconditional Love

If we focus on the teachings of Jesus, Sai Baba, and the other ascended masters, we will find ourselves in a much better place than if we follow those institutions secretly guided by money and control.

Conclusion

My hope is that this book has changed your life and provided you an insight into the modalities of divine healing, as well as the factors that raise and lower your vibration. It's important to set your goals to achieve Christ Consciousness; a high vibrational, unconditionally loving, fruitful life, where you are living in what I call, heaven on earth. Living in this space attracts abundance in every facet of your life, including connecting with your soul mate, enjoying a full flourishment of relationships, and succeeding in life's endeavors. This will provide you with absolute joy.

It's important that anything you do with your gifts—be it creating websites, writing letters, teaching others—that you do this yourself. Do not subcontract out, but rather, sow your energy into the function you're performing. The reason that Ginelle creates and manages our website is to imprint it with her high vibrational energy rather than infuse it with the energy of someone we don't know.

If you have a talent, take it out there and allow others to experience joy or upliftment as the fulfillment of your gift.

It's no use just talking about prayers and being in a high vibrational state, you have to live it, and shift your whole life to accomplish it.

Live an amazing life!

Love your life!

Love and be grateful for your home and everyone you come in contact with!

Be thankful for being alive in this great time!

Testimonials

Carol's Story

On a summer day in 2012 at the annual Chicago Health Expo I stood in a packed room feeling waves of energy run down my body. Thus began my association with Chris Macklin as he did energy work on the entire audience at once. Following his presentation, I asked about treating Lyme disease which I'd had for 35 years and he explained that we could only go as fast as my immune system would allow without causing discomfort or die off symptoms. As it turns out that's not fast enough for me, because I wanted this out of my life decades ago, but maybe I'm alive to learn some patience. My major problem for the last ten years, while I've tried to treat Lyme infections, was an extremely over reactive immune system that produced migraines, hives or pain, in response to any antibiotics, medications, herbs, chemicals and to many foods. Over the years as my health moved along on a downhill slide, more problems developed; cataracts and floaters appeared in my eyes, sinus infections came around all winter, anxiety/memory problems and stabbing muscle pains were frequent, arthritis invaded and a lack of motivation was ever present. I tried amphetamines for that, but guess what, more migraines.

Listening to experts and constant reading has led me to consume mountains of supplements, gallons of camel milk, sea veggies and even kale, which I swear, will never make it off my list of vile foods. Of course as I got more desperate I ventured into acupuncture, Nambudripod Allergy Elimination Technique, cell therapy, hormone replacement, biophoton treatment, rife sessions, electromagnetic therapy, methylation supplements, homeopathics, essential oils, infrared sauna and prayers. All were helpful but none were a cure.

Before Chris, I had decided the most I could hope for would be to treat infections minimally, detox slowly, continue small amounts of supplements and wait until someone could find a better way to treat me. In the meantime, my low energy meant spending most days at home and though I looked quite normal I barely had a life.

Since we began, Chris has been working to eliminate Borrelia first and that should be gone in about a month, co-infections will be next, then DNA reprogramming. Already the diminished load on my system has translated into more energy and stabbing pains are gone. Thoughts about some plans for the future are even creeping in -unbelievable! In a few more months I expect to eat all the spicy tasty foods I've avoided for years, clean out the garage, organize paperwork and paint again. I suppose exercise and yard work should be on my list too. I hardly remember what a normal productive day looks like but now I hope to have many of those soon.

Gracie and Family

"Life is a journey not a destination." - Frost

My History

For the past years I've been on a spiritual journey. I was born into Catholicism, I both respect and honor my religion but I'm not practicing like I would like to. My beliefs have molded who I am today; I'm a strong and caring person. Life after a broken marriage has been very trying for me as well as for my children. Poor kids! A hard life was a normal life. You see, I was totally dependent upon him. We were abundant for being such a young couple. I was such a fool in love; I blame it on my youth and being too trusting. My ex-husband Frank cheated in one of the worst unimaginable ways. I couldn't believe what just happened! What did I do? After the dust settled and all was confirmed I decided not to stand by and watch. I took my children by their little hands and we walked away as he cursed at me. He was so angry and yelled out that I would never amount to anything. Nobody would ever want me with so many kids. I'd never have a car, a home, happiness, any money. I'd be in constant debt. If I took a man into my home he would molest our kids. Frank threatened if I got child support involved he would take the kids and I would never find them in his native country of Mexico. Hearing those last two statements was enough for me. I never pressed legal charges and I quietly faded away. I knew by leaving my home I was walking right into a hardship I've never known. I walked away from a comfortable life; I was alone and afraid. I sought prayer and healings from my church and retreats but nothing seemed to help. I was still feeling afraid: still experiencing financial setbacks. I was always sick, always had this drained and tired feeling. If it wasn't my headaches, it was my stomach or it was my lower back. I tried so hard to be optimistic and to stay positive for my kids but anything and everything was so draining. Months later, I learned the woman my ex got involved with, practices the dark arts. Just the thought of that was so overwhelming for me, so I ignored it and didn't want to believe it.

I believe last year was the worst for me. I suddenly began losing my hair. I was taking pain aids just to start my day…I was so tired when I woke up. When I came home from work, I would take more pain medication just to fall asleep. This became an everyday routine, all year long. One financial set back after another, I was beginning to believe everything he told me was really happening. I couldn't catch a break no matter what I did or didn't do. I was going through all the motions…I was numb, just existing. At this point I was ready to throw in the towel.

The Booking

October 2013, I came across a healing conference and I decided I would attend. I noticed individual healings were being offered by Mr. Macklin. I felt compelled to book the healing; strangely I knew this is what I needed. I can't explain it but somehow I could feel how compassionate he was.

My Sister Ester

I booked the healing for myself but curiously the thought of my sister wouldn't stop and I couldn't understand why. After about two weeks of this, I decided to bring her along and I convinced myself this was meant for her. I love my sister dearly, she's genuinely kind to all and wears her heart on her sleeve. You see my sister had a stroke a few years ago and is currently dealing with a divorce and all its heartaches. Ester is a vulnerable person by nature. When her marriage began to fail, her whole world stopped. I truly felt she wouldn't live past Christmas. As we were driving to the conference my sister kept falling asleep, she was mumbling, she was dizzy, and then she'd wake up to nausea (she doesn't drink). I was so scared and regretful of bringing her along; I thought she was going to die. Twice I woke her up and told her we were turning back because she was getting worse. With all her might she yelled out to keep on driving because she needs to get healed. Poor girl, her eyes were tightly shut because her head was spinning. Inexplicably, when we arrived at the Queen Mary all of what she was experiencing came to a halt. This was either a coincidence or this was supernatural. At last, we meet Mr. Macklin. I can't explain but the second I met him I knew he would make everything better. When my sister met Mr. Macklin he visually scanned her from head to toe and began to name off all that ails her. Ester turned to me with this puzzled look on her face and asked me if I told him about her? I was reassuring her that the both of us are meeting him for the first timer. Macklin just smiled. This was so amazing he can see what was causing her dis-ease as he put it. My sister is 49 years old and has aged so much since her stroke; she's like an unhealthy 60 year old woman.

Then there's Katherine

My daughter is the youngest of 5, she is beautiful, she is kind, she is smart, and she is a teenager. I wasn't aware but both Katherine and I were experiencing the empty nest syndrome. Her three older sisters and her brother Joshua whom she grew close to in the past year had all graduated and began full time jobs and or school. My daughters fiancé passed away last year; he was a constant fixture in our home and she loved him like a brother. Katherine wakes up to everyone scrambling out of the house and comes home to an empty house. Before, there was always some sort of ruckus going on but someone was always home. As for me, she sees me when I came home from work for about 3 hrs then I have to turn in. We do things on my weekends off but she's alone most of the time. She wasn't sleeping, her stomach constantly ached but oddly she was always hungry, the headaches, the nightmares, the constant thoughts of unworthiness and her back was always hurting. Katherine wasn't allowed to date and here's why; she didn't keep her end of the bargain concerning school and there were consequences. One afternoon, (I'll never forget the look on her face) Katherine told me her boyfriend broke up with her. "I'm like what boyfriend?" She was very upset to say the least so I began making plans to go to Disneyland thinking this would cheer her up. Katherine made a comment, "I'm glad I didn't do what I wanted to after all! I asked what she meant and she just smiled. She wouldn't tell me. Katherine was in therapy the next day and boy was she angry. She began acting out at school and soon after I received a message about her behavior. When I asked her what was going on, she broke down screaming that she wanted to slit her wrists and that I just didn't understand. She didn't want to be here, she had no purpose and she wasn't good at anything. I was afraid she would hurt herself and eventually I would fall asleep. Katherine was admitted for a 72 hr. hold and now she really hated me. She told me I gave up on her and I abandoned her. She claimed I threw her away with the real crazy people. I was at a loss; I was unable to help my baby. I was told she had abandonment issues since it wasn't gradual and this gave her anxieties.

My Healing

This truly has been an amazing life changing experience. I had a total of 7 healings yet I noticed after each healing the loss of fear felt was so empowering. I'm 5'2" and I felt invincible, I felt as if I were a 6'5" super hero! I understood if this is what it feels like…I can't wait until my healing is over! This is going to be awesome! I believed that if my life was going to improve I had to participate 100%. At this point in my life this was a sink or swim moment. Being consistent with the prayers while remaining positive with my surroundings was the hardest thing I've ever chosen to follow through with. I had to change my way of thinking as well as the way I verbalized my thoughts. Two words have been removed from my vocabulary - hopefully and maybe. I now say, "Good things will happen to me no matter what situation I find myself experiencing." I noticed everything started to fall into place. The more I said the prayers the more the heaviness dissipated all around me. I noticed the negative people at work stay away from me and that makes me so happy. It's like my eyes have been opened, I not only feel tall I walk taller. I wake up ready for work. My hair is growing again. My breathing has changed, it's much deeper and I don't feel scared. My thoughts aren't so scrambled and fear based, I can focus. I see the vibrancy in each color, at times I have to blink twice to make sure I'm seeing what I'm seeing. I have answers for questions I don't have personal knowledge about but it's like I have already been there or I've experienced it. It was almost as if old wisdom is re-emerging if that makes any sense. My interests have changed, what was important to me is no longer. Life is so relaxed and it feels so good not to worry. I'm not afraid to move beyond the box I was confined to. Strangely, all of this feels right; like this is the way it should have been years ago. My six senses have exploded; nothing is normal anymore. I've learned how to identify and ward off spiritual attacks. With all sincerity I can say that there is no looking back. I don't ever want to return to that dark place I was in for so many years. I will not allow any negativity to hurt me again. After experiencing the warm sinking peaceful feeling that is so awesome...I always want to be there. It feels so safe and I know I'm not alone. My only regrets are that I didn't seek help sooner.

Mr. Macklin our Angel on Earth

The day we first met Mr. Macklin we felt so comfortable, there was a pleasant welcoming feeling about him. It was like he exuded virtuousness almost on a holy level. It was powerful. I felt like a child that was finally safe and nothing could touch me now. I see a man, but if I were to close my eyes he feels like and would be a holy man. After one of my healings I told him my daughter had suicidal thoughts and he immediately made arrangements for her healing. I couldn't believe it! He offered to heal her...he made time for her and he was willing to save her. He was booked far in advance but he made time to save my daughter's soul. He is a noble man. There was an incident that occurred right after my 3rd healing - I had a spiritual attack of excruciating pain. I wasn't aware it was an attack. I had taken pain killers all day and nothing worked. I remember reminding my daughter about her healing coming up in a few minutes when I thought of one of the prayers. I didn't have it nearby so I focused on hearing Mr. Macklin's voice recite his prayer...God is my witness the pain stopped immediately! It was incredible! I couldn't believe what just happened. This was intense! I've had 2 prior esoteric healings, both of which the results were very temporary, nothing like this. After the first healing we received from Mr. Macklin, it would be days later we were still flying hi in the clouds. It's an everlasting feeling of happiness, optimism and Unconditional Love... I just wanted to bust!

Three Lives are Saved

My sister Ester had given up and was on the verge of surrendering to her illnesses. He's removed the black cloud hanging over her and has breathed life back into her. She would get around using a walker but now she forgets to use it because she doesn't need it anymore. Her excruciating hip and arm pain is gone. Ester is so much happier now that her pain is almost gone. She can't believe how quick her health is improving and she's very opinionated too if I might add. She isn't 100% but she's getting there. She's optimistic and she's alive. Ester no longer has death on her mind she is so grateful to Mr. Macklin that she has a new lease on life.

Katherine's suicidal thoughts have ceased, she wonders if it will come back. She has faith and trusts in God as she was a non-believer. Katherine is able to distinguish real sadness from bad sadness (she knows the feeling) and will not allow those evil thoughts to take over again. Katherine is a work in progress and is learning to use the prayers. She can't believe how close she came to giving up on herself and understands what was behind it. Katherine is so giggly now; she's a child again and is happy. Katherine likes to talk about her healing but gets the chills just thinking about it, she's still perplexed about what she experienced but she came out a believer. I have my daughter once again and every day we are closer.

Me? Well I've learned so much and I've witnessed unbelievable things during our healings. That half dead person with chronic pain is gone. My kids have the mother they should have had years ago but it's never too late. I'm enjoying my kids and my new life without pain. I'm often visited by humming birds which is such a heavenly blessing. My whole world has been turned right side up and now I have to catch up to it. I can't express how profound the healing and the prayers are. I am so grateful! I may not have everything my ex cursed me with but I am confident I will have exactly all of that in the near future. I am of God and I am grounded to the earth!

Mr. Macklin has been so kind, generous and patient with us. I'm honored to have met him as well as to have been able to receive his healings and blessings. I will forever be indebted to this noble man we know as Mr. Macklin.

God Bless You and your family! May the light of God forever shine upon you!

Paul's Story

During the 1990s I first started experiencing symptoms which in the last several years, became an extremely difficult physical and emotional struggle. It evolved to the point where I would question my sanity and even my will to live. Initially, I noticed bumps on my face and eventually I discovered that these bumps originated directly by my whiskers. So, I would use tweezers to pull out the whiskers from my face. The hair shaft would be coated in a whitish or clear substance like if you pulled out a fence post from the ground that was set in cement. This only happened periodically in the 90s, maybe three or four whiskers every couple of months. Nothing alarming, even though it was puzzling. After about five years, this progressed to the point where my neck was covered with these abnormal whiskers, until they eventually progressed up from my neck and chin towards my cheeks.

I tried numerous techniques to try and rid myself of these abnormal whiskers. I scrubbed, steamed and soaked until I began to realize that I was dealing with something that was like a curse. I felt invaded. Something was infiltrating my skin and apparently there was nothing that I could do about it.

I spent many nights obsessively splashing water on my face, pulling whiskers out…trying to find even the most modest amount of relief from what seemed like torture from within. Also, at regular intervals, I would also get various sores on different parts of my face, usually it would take one to two weeks for them to heal. It was a nuisance, but, manageable. Not overly alarming. Just something that was similar to what I had dealt with since my teenage years when I suffered from a moderate case of acne.

The annoying part of the process was that it always seemed like my face would clear up. Then within a week or two, the next round of blemishes would start again. A continual cycle of having to battle against whatever was causing this to happen. I was constantly wondering why a person in his 30s would have to be subjected to the symptoms of a teenager. At times it was emotionally and mentally exhausting. It absolutely had a negative impact on my social life and my mental well being. I was never able to develop a consistent pattern of having a normal appearance.

Then, approximately five years ago I started experiencing the sensation that something was growing or crawling on my face and the whisker problem continued. I was trying every type of substance I could think of to try and rid myself of the physical and emotional trauma that I was experiencing. I bought a facial steamer, thinking that I could dissolve away the material. That didn't work!

I would obsessively splash isopropyl alcohol on my face in an extreme, but, ultimately futile attempt to control the indescribable sensation covering my face. I would go to work and take facial scrub, soap and alcohol to use during the day. By the end of a very long day (12-14 hours) I would have the sensation of something "growing" over my entire face.

This small problem that had begun about 10 years earlier had become a daily struggle. I would find myself up for hours and hours during the night trying to get relief from the whisker problem. Obsessively picking and pulling out my whiskers with tweezers. At times even falling asleep while standing up in front of a mirror as I was trying to rid myself of these invaders that were causing me such emotional trauma.

I was incessantly searching the Internet trying to find out what was wrong with me. Seeing if other people were experiencing the same strange symptoms. I found out that I was not alone. That other individuals were having similar problems and were struggling with it just like me. At least I didn't feel alone, even though I lived alone and had no one to turn to for guidance or support. I tried to go to a couple of doctors.

One treated me like I had teenage acne. Of course, that didn't help. Another, presented with physical and photographic evidence of my troubles, immediately printed out a lengthy article on delusions of parasitosis. He sent me on my way with a look of sympathy for my mental instability and the advice to go see a psychologist. Fortunately, the anger and frustration that accompanied that diagnosis did not fully manifest until days later. There is no telling what I might have said to that person if I had immediately processed the demeaning and absurd diagnosis.

In 2010 I used an Indian healing formula internally. About six weeks after I began, I started to get extremely large scabs on my face. Long, bloody "creatures" would pop out of my skin when I picked the scabs. Some were about 1 1/2" long.

It was terrifying! Horrifying! I was not able to comprehend what was happening to me. I felt like I was living in a real life horror movie. It took an extreme amount of mental gymnastics to maintain my sanity. I could not leave my house for almost a month due to the fact that about half of my face was covered in horrendously large scabs. When I was finally able to go to the store, I wore a hoodie sweatshirt with the drawstring pulled tight so I could hide both sides of my face. I'm sure the security cameras were very interested in my movements. The scabs eventually cleared after I stopped taking the Indian formula. However, that was not the end of my problems. I would get sores on my face, about the size of a quarter and sometimes bigger, that would ooze a somewhat sticky substance. My whiskers continued to be coated in the material. About three years ago I started using a concoction that helped remove the substances from my face. Unimaginable things came out of my skin; tightly wound fiber clusters, globs of material like firm cottage cheese, long, stringy white and pink substances. Also, some of my whiskers were deformed when I pulled them out. Some looking like a blade of grass, others like a palm leaf. Very long thin fibers came out of my face. Sometimes they were straight, other times I would get clumps that looked like a foot of black thread coiled up in a ball. The emotional impact was immense. I wish I had a nickel for each time I said to myself, "I can't take this anymore."

For over a year I couldn't go more than three or four days without having to put one or two bandages on my face to cover up some sort of problem. Most of time those bandages had to stay on for at least a week or two, sometimes even longer. My life was ruined. I couldn't work because I never knew what was going to come out of my face. Many times it was embarrassing to be seen in public. Fortunately, I heard about Christopher Macklin. If it wasn't for his Divine Healing methods I'm not sure I would be around today to write this testimonial because I frequently wondered why I had any reason to live.

Before meeting Christopher, I literally had no hope. I was on the brink of giving up because a solution to my problem seemed impossible. However, I knew from the very first session that I had the amazingly good fortune to finally find a person who could actually help me. A person who could give me hope! A person who could rescue me from my despair! Christopher is so caring, giving, and understanding. I could tell that he is driven by his desire to help others. I felted blessed!

During the sessions the sensations going through my body were amazing. I felt like I was being scrubbed from the inside; that the source of my problem was being attacked and eliminated. It was as if the unwanted material was being purged from my body. After all the years of trying every possible solution, I found my ability to see the future, to see something other than my demise. The progress has been steady and extremely noticeable. Areas of my face that have been bothering me for years have disappeared. Due to the elimination of the substances below my skin, my facial structure has changed. I am starting to look like myself again. Also, the results have completely changed my outlook on life. I feel like I can be a functioning member of society again!

Before, every day was a massive challenge just to get up the courage to go out in public. Without Christopher Macklin, I don't know how much longer I would have been able to exist in that state of darkness and depression. Finally, after so many struggles, so many attempts at correcting this problem, so many nights of questioning how much longer I could cope with my situation, I was blessed with the one person who could change my life.

Darkness has been replaced by a beaming bright light.... And it is beautiful!

Words will never be able to adequately convey my gratitude and appreciation to the incredibly wonderful person named Christopher Macklin.

Sarah's Story

The Brave New World!

It has been almost a year and a half since I was beaten with a small board resulting in a final blow to the back of the head. Several doctors later, the diagnosis was Post- Concussive Syndrome and PTSD with a twist. I was thrust into a totally different world. One in which hearing and light sensitivities changed my life dramatically.

Every tiny sound was so loud I could barely stand to be in my body. It was like having an out of control radio strapped to your head with broken volume controls playing all of the channels simultaneously full blast. Of course, your hands would be tied so that you could not remove it. In the beginning days, I would dash around the apartment to locate where the loud, scary sound was coming from. One night the extremely loud bellows sound, like one used to stoke a blast furnace, turned out to be my calico cat Gwendalyn snoozing away on her high perch. Watching TV was almost impossible due to sirens, fast car and kid noises.

Then there were the headaches, the shaking and the exhaustion. Three different varieties of headaches including lightening, all day camp outs and the gypsies wandered around my head constantly. Everything triggered the headaches, shaking and the exhaustion that quickly always followed. No relief was in sight.

Sounds, bright lights, strangers, being out in the world by myself, made driving no longer possible. It took several months before a driver found me so that I could escape the sounds of gardeners, lawn mowers and blowers. I don't know how I made it to Christmas!

Welcome to my Physical Reality!

Now what? How can I possibly live like this?

The first few months are a blur now. At first, all I was able to do was hold a cat and take pictures while it was snoring on my lap. I could not drive. My apartment was full of extremely loud, very frightening noises that constantly triggered headaches, shaking and instant exhaustion. Being in a grocery store was nearly impossible. Driving was out of the question for almost a year.

Then Heaven started sending me aid. Friends suggested ear plugs and sent Indian headache salve. I had to buy a new T.V. that would accommodate headsets. In order to survive kitchen noises, I ate with plastic utensils, covered the counter with rubber matting and put it in between the dishes in the cupboard. A friend put rubber dots on the cupboard doors to mute the sound when they closed. She went through the apartment using WD-40 to cancel out squeaking doors and all manner of hinges. I had to leave my apartment in order to wash clothes. So, I rarely washed because being out of my apartment triggered the shaking and panic attacks. I was not able to use a vacuum cleaner and ended giving away the large one that made machine noises in exchange for a small Dyson. The squeak refused to leave my big, comfy recliner and so it had to find a new home. The new chair has no moving parts and thus does not talk. There have been many adjustments. I am grateful for all of the people who have come to offer assistance in uncountable ways.

I appreciate you all!

Just becoming functional to this degree required a tremendous amount of work, patience and many months of problem solving. Currently driving is only possible on the best and strongest energy days. Just writing this is causing some tiredness. I am going to have to stop now and rest.

The Magic of Macklin!

When he entered my world this fall, the noise sensitivity and nervous system overstimulation were the biggest priorities. In over a year, there had been no change. No matter what I tried, there was no relief. The sounds were barely tolerable using the highest decibel ear plugs simultaneously with a Bose Noise Cancellation Headset. Watching TV was still challenging and meant using the mute button often even while wearing ear plugs.

As he began to work with me, I noticed immediately that there was a shift in the nervous system tension. Every few days at the beginning of our sessions he would ask me what had changed. I would always think to myself, "Christopher, are you nuts! There has been no change to the sound levels in a year. You are expecting changes in three days?! How can this possibly be?" Well you have to understand that between Christopher Macklin and Heaven, everything is possible. He expects it and it happens! Macklin Magic!

The days melted into weeks and months. Much to my surprise, I would always have a new success to report. As the nervous system continued to balance, I am now able to drive on certain days to local places. How long I can stay is anyone's guess, at least I can get there and back. On most days I am able to be in my apartment without earplugs and that is huge. Grocery shopping has been an insurmountable event. Now, for a short period of time, I am actually able to survive the announcements and loud music using only earplugs without becoming a hot shaking mess. Sounds like the refrigerator, clothes washer and dryer are coming into more normal ranges and are far more manageable than ever before.

My gratitude goes out to Mr. Macklin for the kindness, caring and love that he gives in his sessions. I highly recommend Macklin Ministries and hold their talents, hard work and dedication in high esteem.

Elliot's Story

Besides the normal every day entity removal (yeah, just like in Ghostbusters but without the storage fee), I have had healing sessions with Chris - remotely, in person & over the phone. All work equally well!

I have had improvement in so many areas. Just to pick one in particular, I've got a scar on the bottom of my left foot. From this 1967 trauma, I underwent a hospital stay complete with a blood transfusion. As a parting gift, I got a cast to wear for almost a year. The coat hanger to scratch with was extra. The scar had barely budged in 47 years... until Chris worked on it.

Right now it has improved and softened to the point where my balance is sometimes actually better with this foot!

Now, add to that, he's fun to work with.
It doesn't get any better than that.
Period!

Michael's Story

This is my True Testimonial!

My name is Michael, I developed an unknown virus around 7 years ago. I first noticed my condition when my body began swelling up like a balloon. My knees started aching to the point where walking was becoming painful and difficult. At the time I thought I had been bitten by a tick, but without a red spot or bulls eye the doctor said it was not the issue. My mom and I traveled all over the East Coast looking for answers, trying all kinds of treatments. Nothing worked and my condition continued to worsen.

Five years passed and my condition was progressing rapidly, to the point of not being able to walk, brush my teeth, dress myself, or eat. My knees froze at a 90 degree angle, locking up, this is the way they stayed. My joints all began to swell, my fingers, my hips, my knees. The last few years my mom has taken care of me because my ex wife wouldn't help. She basically left me for dead!

My mom was researching remedies and answers when she found Christopher. He has helped me tremendously. I have regained mobility in my joints to a certain point. I have more energy with every session. I can now stand on my feet again. It's been 2 years since I've walked!

Due to Christopher's help I am hoping to get on my feet again and play with my 8 year old child. I believe as long as you believe in the healing and the power of the Holy Spirit, it is possible for anything. It is possible through the word, works of Christ, and God to heal and help me find my way back to the mobility of walking again.
Always have Faith, and the love of Christ!

Thank you!

Brandon's Story

Fitness is my Life!

I still will be thankful for the session and healing I received. Over the last three years, I've had pain in the right arm from an accident that broke my wrist in two places. I needed surgery, which involved a lot of cutting and a lot of metal put in place of bone. The pain began within around a year after the surgery and magnified quickly. Until the point of icing my arm everyday caused thinking of other options for work, since I work in a gym. Day to day activities involve lifting heavy objects and helping people by demonstrating exercises. I was at that point when sleep didn't come easy. If I did manage to fall asleep, one turn in bed and I was back up. Sleep was done for that night!

Now things are much better! The pain in my arm is gone. Work is much easier and comfortable. As soon as I started my sessions, I could feel things going on in the places of my arm that had the most pain and discomfort. Within a couple of months it was gone! I still am amazed that the pain went from every hour to now nothing at all.

I am positive now that fitness can continue to be the passion in my life. This is all because of the healing I received.

Thank you!

Stacey's Story

I was diagnosed with fibromyalgia about two years ago. Anxiety had become completely uncontrollable and severe depression overshadowed my entire life. I had extreme fatigue and pain all day, every day. I could barely get out of bed. I went to several doctors and specialists. Had so many tests performed: blood labs, x-rays, nerve tests, and a MRI. Nothing was abnormal!

Then came the treatments. Medications piled on top of medications. At one time I was taking 8 medications at once and nothing helped. In fact I was taking medications to help with the side effects of medications. I was literally being medicated for being medicated. This went on for another year and nothing changed except my bank account drained from so many visits and meds to replace meds. Needless to say, I certainly learned a lot about the insurance and medical industry. For a last ditch effort, I was recommended to a pain management clinic. I couldn't believe this was my last hope. But it wasn't!

Then I met Christopher!

I can't really express in words what my experience with him was like. I just don't think there are words in our vocabulary to describe it. Miraculous? Extraordinary? Any word is a grave understatement. I guess all I can say is that he healed me with the Divine Healing Love of the Creator.

So to all those who have been told you have fibromyalgia, go see Christopher! You know the drugs aren't working. They aren't really getting to the core of the problem. Christopher healed me physically and emotionally.

I feel whole again!

Sharlene's Story

Living in the Twilight Zone

Oozing sores! Open holes where bugs crawl under the skin! Strings pushing their way through your eyes, your teeth, your ears! This is a little of the living hell I have experienced for far too long. I am not alone! There are hundreds of thousands of us here in the United States and all over the world. Many can no longer physically or mentally endure. They simply find a way to end their lives. After all, it isn't as though you are living any longer. Some don't have a choice; they die from isolation, hopelessness and this unexplained illness. I am an ordinary person with an extraordinary life. This is part of my story. You will probably doubt what I will tell you but hopefully God will help you to see that it is true.

I was blessed throughout my life because I always had a great faith in God. I always believed. Many miracles have happened throughout my 60 years on this earth. My childhood years were difficult as they are with most, but I always had a mother who loved me. If you have someone who really loves you have what you need. Graduating from high school at only 17, I boasted an engagement ring on my finger by age 18. In those days, most girls planned to pursue a career in homemaking. I married at age 18 but didn't become a mother until I was 26 years old. I gave birth to an amazing son. Life was pretty normal until at age 35when I was diagnosed with breast cancer.

My family was told to prepare for a funeral within the next 6 months. Doctors placed me on strong doses of chemotherapy and also a long treatment with radiation therapy. At first I refused the treatment but after considering my 9 year old son living life without a mom, I made myself put those poisons into my body every day. I always wore my hair long. Everyday I'd watch and wait for it to fall out. It happened all at once. I will never forget standing in the shower one day washing my hair and finding my hands full of clumps of hairs. It was horrifying! My beautiful hair and breast were gone. I wondered if I would open my eyes to the world and not think "I have cancer."

I talked to God all the time. I felt so loved by my family and for the loved they bestowed on me. Actually, I felt grateful for this horrible experience because I now really appreciate life and every little thing in it. It was as if I had woken up into a new world, one in which nothing was to be taken for granted. The good china was longer to be used only on special occasions. Vacations wouldn't be put off for years until we could pay the way! Appreciate every day because it may be your last!

Embracing life became a real priority. I made a sincere prayer to God one night as I lay there thinking about how blessed I was. I sobbed thinking of all the women who had gone though this with no one to hold them! No one to support them! I thought of all the people who suffer all over the world. I thought of the animals and the planet in need of so much help. And the prayer I made to God was a heartfelt request for God to use me as an instrument to bring love and healing to this planet and its people. The prayer was sincere and I believe it was answered because my heart felt like it would burst with joy.

Eventually the day did come when I didn't wake up in the morning thinking "Is it back?" The cancer went away but my health was still not good. I couldn't seem to get past the anemia problems. Blister like pimples began to erupt on my arms and legs. These itched intensely, worse than poison ivy or chicken pox. Even more troubling was my inability to sleep at night. I would sit up all night long, itching so severely that I just wanted to scream. It was embarrassing to go to the grocery store because of the lesions on my arms and legs. These dime sized craters were oval shaped with thick borders. The tops looked as though they were sealed with amber.

My 20 year old marriage began to deteriorate. I went to doctors and a dermatologist who gave me ointments which didn't help at all. When I showed the dermatologist the blister akin to chicken pox, he followed through with a biopsy. He found nothing and insinuated that it was in my head. I finally went to a country doctor who was fresh out medical school. He suspected that I might have Systemic Lupus Erythematosus (LUPUS). The DNA results came back positive for SLE so we assumed the symptoms on my skin were connected to that disease. Later I would be diagnosed also with Raynaud's, Jorgen's, Fibromyalgia, Restless Leg Syndrome and more!

As the next years passed, my health, my home and my husband were all gone. My dreams and body felt broken. I went into a severe depression. After having lesions on my body for over 2 years, they instantly disappeared as if having distance from the stress of my relationship had healed me. After two more surgeries, I finally found a very minimal paying job. I went back to college to complete a counseling degree. I wanted to help others more than anything.

There were many little miracles that took place for me and oddly enough my son and I were now happier and more peaceful than we had ever been. The health problems continued including severe migraine headaches. Just the same, I forged ahead in life with a great strength and joy. Feeling a purpose to my life!

After graduating, I worked for a few years in the VA. Then God lead me to the great NW, to the Seattle area. It was a scary experience for a girl who had never been away from home. The great Northwest is more than great! I love its scenery, its climate and its wonderful open and accepting people. It felt as though it had always been my home. I loved my new job too.

During my workday in 2001, I was injured in a hit and run auto accident. It was a very difficult time. I went through many therapies including a stay in a rehabilitation pain clinic. I became very ill. My fever shot up and a large black spot the size of a quarter had grown inside my cheek. I was sent to the doctor who was puzzled by what he called a necrosis in my mouth. I was sent for further investigation. My face was very swollen. It looked like I had gained one hundred pounds.

This was a turning point in my life...the return of the strange illness and the beginning of a true nightmare! A large paisley shaped lesion formed at the base of my skull. In the shape were small growths. It itched enough to keep you from relaxing, sleeping and functioning. It grew larger and larger. I went from dermatologist to dermatologist who purported that it was psoriasis, eczema etc. The strange lesion spread upward through the scalp pulling in the long hairs and creating cyst like structures underneath. Over and over I went to the dermatologist, took their antibiotics and shots of cortisone to my head to no avail. I pleaded with them to help! They kept telling me not to touch it. It was unbearable! It is hard to describe to you, but it felt like something moving inside of your skin. Underneath there was growth going on. A system of tubes, roots, and fibers were setting up a network. I tried not touching it. That was the wrong thing to do! It just kept growing and setting up its network. My face became very swollen again. My head and scalp became completely misshapen. I went from doctor to doctor but nothing worked. Most of the dermatologists became downright nasty to me as if I was somehow responsible for this condition. They had no idea what I was experiencing! The horror of feeling something growing under your skin. That play "Little Shop of Horrors" kept coming to mind.

Other strange things started to manifest. When I took a bath, I would find the tub full of balls of lint and sometimes spiders. I also kept finding spiders and webs in my car even though I did not park under trees. My hair brush was full of lint balls even though it was cleaned weekly and my hair was falling out all over the place. When I stood in front of the bathroom mirror (a large mirror that covered half the wall) my hair would stand straight up as if there was an electrical charge pulling it. It would dance back and force. Bizarre! When I walked past street lights they would often just blow out. Red white and blue fibers were all over my apartment. The itchy lesions returned again this time everywhere. Such a misery cannot be adequately described nor would I want you to understand this pain. At that point the hair on my head was being sucked into the oozing craters on my scalp and encased in a gooey clear substance that was like a super glue. I was unable to find help in the medical community. All their medications and all their diagnosis's seemed to be inadequate.

Finally I looked on the internet for skin diseases and itching which lead me to a site for the "Morgellons Research Foundation". This organization was based out of the University of Oklahoma where research was being conducted on Morgellons. More than 14,000 families had registered there whose symptoms were similar to mine. The Morgellons Foundation hired a neuroscientist named Randy Wymore to examine samples from patients. With the aid of the Tulsa Police Dept. a forensics team was able to conclude the Morgellons fibers were not a match for any know fibers here on earth. So where do they come from? Further, Vitaly Citovisky, Professor of Biochemistry at Stony Brook University in NY compared blood samples from Morgellons volunteers to non Morgellons volunteers. All samples from Morgellons volunteers where positive for Agrobacteria Tumefactions. Agrobacteria Tumefactions is inserted into plants for the purpose of genetic modification. It is used in GMO (Genetically Modified Organisms) food and the creation of vaccines. Citovisky recommended a further study. Many years later Citovisky would recant and deny his clearly written paper.

It was comforting to finally have a name to pin on this nightmare. Even more comforting was the thought that I was not alone. As I would find out later there were hundreds of thousands of us all over the world. The largest concentration of people with Morgellons are in the U.S especially in Texas, California and Florida. Other sufferers had posted their stories on the website. These were heartbreaking to read. I couldn't imagine infants and small children, dogs, cats and horses all having to suffer with this pain and rejection. Also, there were letters from government officials requesting the investigation of Morgellons by the CDC. Even Barack Obama requested further study by the CDC. During this period of time, 2006, the CDC listed Morgellons as an unknown dermopathy. It also said it related closely to Lyme disease. As far as I know everyone with Morgellons has Lyme disease. Morgellons was listed under its National Center for Zoonotic Vector-

Borne and Enteric Disease. It had been listed and transferred to the Army's Bioterrorism Unit. Vectors generally refer to arthropods. Enteric diseases are bacterial and viral infections of the gastrointestinal tract. After keeping this Morgellons study for years, the Army reported no information but instead released the study to a medical insurance group, Kaiser Permanente, who had recently defrauded the U.S. government.

Doctors continued to treat us like we were delusional even though delusional parasitosis is extremely rare. This is a label that was cast upon the Morgellons community without any real proof. Along the way, I have found a few good and open-minded doctors who are compassionate. Most I have met make you feel that you are less than human...invisible. The fact that most morgies become overweight and lose their teeth further contributes to the perception that the patient is simply not educated or healthy. This is simply not true. There are actually quite a few doctors and nurses who have Morgellons. Marc Neumann of Germany did do some survey of a large number of sufferers all over the world. His website is www.Morgellons-research.org.

My condition continued to worsen. I kept regular bi-weekly appointments with the Head of Dermatology at the University of WA. I was in agony. There were strange spaghetti like strands growing under my skin on my derriere. The Dr. had a group of his colleagues to set up cameras to film the area. This was very embarrassing. It felt like hard uncooked strains the size of spaghetti noodles. All totaled there were 7 biopsies done which revealed nothing but plant material. The back of my head became so inflamed and painful that the mere wind blowing on it hurt. The Dr. phoned the burn unit of the hospital and they sent over a Dr. to evaluate my scalp. They said that I had the equivalent of 3rd degree burns. There was no real way to bandage this area but they gave me jelly like pads that could be laid on the raw tissue. All anyone would have to do was to look at me to determine that what I was experiencing wasn't in my mind. The Dr. in Dermatology preceded to take it upon himself to write letters to all of my doctors informing them that I thought that I had Morgellons and that surely meant that I was suffering from DOP (delusions of parasitosis). This reaction of disbelief continues with most doctors whom Morgellons patients see. It would seem to me that they are the delusional ones. Because he had written this letter to the other doctors, it felt quite odd! No shocking! He had contacted another doctor, an internist, at Bastyr Medical Center. He asked her to telephone me. When the call came in from Dr. H, I knew nothing of her or the call she had received. We talked and Dr. H told me that she had many patients with Morgellons. She scheduled an appointment. I was thrilled. Her visit provided me with an official diagnosis of Morgellons and Lyme with its confections. She treated me with respect and compassion. I was given 3 heavy duty medications. One was for leprosy and one was for tuberculosis. I stayed on these for several years. Another medication?

My anemia continued to persist. You can't go places because you have to stay in close proximity of the bathroom. The itching and crawling in your eyes and ears stop you from getting to sleep. I even had to pull off the road when driving because of strings moving in my ears or sharp pains in the eyes as the strings come through the eye. It feels like you have been stuck with a pin. Those of us who have had cancer or shingles know about pain. We know how to fight. Morgellons pain and discomfort supersedes it all. It feels like it was made to destroy our spirit. We cannot let it win. One night I almost let it win. My face was covered in hundreds of lesions and swelled 3 times it size. I could feel the crawling sensation on and under my skin. The itching was so extreme. It would not let up. Add to that a migraine headache, sciatica, back and neck pain. You have the picture. I felt I couldn't take anymore. I'd reached the bottom of the pit. I fell down on the floor and began to pray out loud. I started to call out all of my blessings one by one. This went on for what seemed like forever until my pain turned to joy. Now whenever I feel I have reached the bottom of the pit, I say "thank you God" and start naming all that I am grateful for.

The head continued to deteriorate creating a huge crater in the back above the base of the neck. During the day, I had gone to the dermatologist closest to where I lived and pleaded with them to do something for me because this area was unbearable. I looked into the opening in the skull by holding a mirror to the back. I could see what appeared to be an intertwined vine from which hung a large pea pod looking thing. They did not even look at the head. They did nothing but recommend that I seek psychiatric evaluation. I realize that they didn't know what to do with me, but they were cold and unfeeling. Previously, they had given me shots of cortisone in my head, removed cysts, tried ointments and medications but none had helped. It was a horrible situation to be in. Around midnight that same evening I found myself in an emergency situation. A blood vessel in the back of my head had burst due to tissue erosion. I was used to bleeding a lot, so I just wrapped a towel around my head to catch the blood and waited for it to stop. I should have realized this wasn't going to stop. Every time I lifted the towel to check if the blood had stopped, it squirted out of the head and all over the walls like a squirt gun. I finally realized that it wasn't stopping which was very frightening. I phoned a nurse friend who lived about 2 minutes away. Although it was about midnight, she arrived in less than 5 minutes. We were quickly at the emergency room door. The emergency room never even asked me for Id, insurance card or anything. They simple phoned back to the Surgeon to meet me in the back room. By the time I was in the back room the Surgeon arrived and removed the towel. She stitched up the blood vessel but it did not last. She commented that the vessels were too dried out. After the second repair it held firm. I was advised to see my Dr. the next day for a follow up. A leather type of patch was applied over the hole. The Surgeon also said that I would need to have additional surgery to cover the opening with permanent plate. There was too much missing tissue for it to close itself up naturally.

With my injuries from the auto accident and the condition of my body from Morgellons, I was forced to give up the job I loved to go on disability. I developed more problems of a neurological nature. With the loss of my job came the loss of my apt. This couldn't have been worse timing. The apartment complex I live in required everyone to move as they were converting all apartments into condos. All tenants must vacate unless they wanted to purchase the condo at a cost of around a half million. Even if you planned to buy one you couldn't avoid moving out until the renovations were done. My disability had not yet been approved complicating a move where income would need to be verified. My son and daughter in law were gracious enough to invite me to move to MA where I could live nearby. They offered to co-sign my lease if necessary. With help from my amazing friends my things were packed and sent on their way. Making the trip proved painful and difficult all around. It took me about 3 weeks to locate a ground floor apt during which time I lived in a hotel. I could not expose my family to Morgellons not knowing if it was contagious or not.

Setting up a doctor network in MA was a challenge too. MA is a progressive state and they already required all of it residents to have health insurance. This meant there was a shortage of primary care doctors. After a long search, I found a nearby primary care doctor and arranged an appointment. I took papers from all my doctors back in WA State. This included the ones that stated I had Lyme Disease and Morgellons. On the initial visit the Dr. informed me that MA did not recognize Lyme disease. It was not recognized by the AMA. I couldn't believe it. Currently, Lyme is considered an epidemic in MA as well as CT. My next appointment which was the actual exam part was cancelled by the doctor's office. The explanation given was that I was too complicated. This reminded me of what my Rheumatologist used to jokingly say that I was his Dr. House patient (a TV show about hard to diagnose patients).

While living in MA I began to photograph the constant exodus of materials that were existing and growing in my body. It felt like I was being devoured. I am a human incubator for who knows what. I see and have filmed embryonic looking samples, tubes the size of straws which grow in my body, insects, fibers, plant life, glitter, photonic crystals, nano- spheres, fabric looking materials and indescribable critter looking things with faces. They grow at an exponential rate. It often feels as though a drill is being forced through my body. There are often 40 to 50 samples exiting per day. I am not alone in the insanity but I choose to record these by film in an effort to validate my reality. It is necessary given that you begin to question your own sanity.

The back of my head healed up but other areas opened up. There was a deep crater that opened up on the side of the head. I began to make to make more contacts with other Morgellons sufferers and their families mainly through a man named Marc Neumann who would end up helping me so much. I am amazed at how many wonderful and giving people are sick with this syndrome. On Wednesdays, I would have a telephone conference with 8 or 9 women who were all Morgies and medical professionals. They told me how the hospitals are full of nurses and other medical people who are Morgellons sufferers. Our group would share ideas, frustrations and treatments. One nurse was so afraid she might lose her 3 year old son. Her husband thought that she was crazy. He left her and filed for custody of the boy. The little boy also was also suffering from the illness. Everyone keeps quiet about what they have for fear of the repercussions. The medical community has turned its back on us.

During our conversations, I was fortunate enough learn of Dr. William Harvey. Dr. Harvey had retired from NASA where he was the Medical Training Director for many years focusing on the medical challenges to humans in space. His years after retirement were devoted to researching unknown infectious diseases. Harvey's goal was to build a clinic where people with Morgellons could go and stay while being treated. Some of the other conference ladies had gone to see Harvey in Colorado and they received testing and also medications thru IV drip. My condition had worsened so much that even though traveling might kill me I was willing to take the chance. A small sample came out of head on the left side that looked very much like a microphone with tiny squares all line up in a row. At that time I did not have my microscope to get a close up look at it so I took it on my journey to see Harvey. During my exam, I gave the sample to the clinic in a baggie and asked them to please identify it and then be sure to return it to me. Harvey sent me to the local hospital for tests. He would use these for a study and a peer reviewed article he was writing. I was not able to stay by myself to receive the IV treatments. Returning home 3 days later, it occurred to me that I shouldn't have left the sample from my head. I did receive medication which included Ivermetin from Dr. Harvey and I was included in his study. Upon my arrival back in MA I called the clinic and asked them to go ahead and send back my head sample. I had a bad feeling about it. Sure enough they informed me that they had lost the sample. Later I would find out the all the samples that others had taken to the clinic had disappeared as well. Those who were able to take the IV treatments had improved greatly which made me regret not finding a way to follow them. Harvey's study revealed many similarities among us. We have anemia, low body temperature and generally thyroid dysfunction to name a few things.

My skin condition continued to worsen to the point where I could hardly get out of bed for an entire year. Sitting and lying down on open wounds is unbearable. It was necessary to shave off all my hair because new sores and wounds kept opening up on the head and the neck. This necessitated my keeping my head covered summer and winter. Pieces of pink yarn like material came out of my body and dropped off of me everywhere I went. This made me hesitant to be in anyone else's environment for fear I'd contaminate them. The CDC finally launched a study into Morgellons in 2008. The Morgellons community was counting on the study to validate our condition and verify whether or not we were safe to be around. We were nervous to be around our families and friends given that the pets and family members sometimes contracted the illness and other times they did not. The CDC study was bogus and the statements made were unclear. They likened our condition to DOP (delusions of parasitosis) but actually said that it was unclear what the cause of Morgellons was or indeed what Morgellons is. They also said that we were not contagious. Hmmm…they don't know what it is but they could confirm it is not contagious??? The community was devastated after waiting for 8 years for the study. Why was a company chosen to do the study who had just been fined for defrauding the US government? The information on the study was released a few months after Dr. William Harvey passed away. Very shortly after the release of the report the main website, Morgellons Research Foundation, was closed down. This had contained invaluable information, articles by doctors, previous reports, and stories from sufferers, photographs and requests from political leaders including Obama for a CDC study. This all disappeared. We were devastated. Our hope to be legitimized in the eyes of our families and the medical community disappeared leaving many of us without hope for medical treatment. The disbelief of families and doctors is the hardest to bare.

A wonderful event happened in February. I became a grandma to a healthy little grandson. It is awesome being a grandparent. I was afraid to go near the baby for fear I'd make him sick. I wouldn't even go in his hospital room. The whole first year, I barely saw the little guy and when I did, it was at a distance. Can you imagine not being able to hug, kiss and hold your grandchild? He is now 4 years old and I have still never held or kissed him. He doesn't get to come into my home either. I do sit next to him now to read a book as long as my skin is covered. This is one of the saddest parts of this affliction. You are afraid to make others sick.

My illness continued to change and express itself in peculiar almost bizarre ways. The most upsetting expression to me was in the insects. I will never forget the day I watched collembolans race across my bathroom floor after exiting my body. Unbelievable! They were lavender in color with sweet faces. Other insecticidal parts surfaced; wasps, wasp wings, cabbage looper worms, moths, and fungal gnats. The ones that were the scariest to me were the spiders. I'm terrified of spiders! But for my photographs, I'd would think that I am mentally ill. Believe you me, I shook with terror as I watched those spider come out of my body!! I also began to see signs of florescent material like photonic crystals, nano spheres, glitter, fibers and samples that looked like 3 week old fetuses. What a creepy show! What horrible pain pulling out tubes the size of drinking straws! I removed one tube and the inside revealed a small green florescent lime bug similar to an aphid with large black eyes. It was very much alive and began to flap its wings. This was all very hard to accept, it doesn't fit into my reality.

Meanwhile, I continued to change my diet eliminating GMO (genetically modified foods). These can change our DNA and have the ability to insert insect DNA into our DNA; plus pesticides are a part of the offering. Over this twenty years I must have tried more than 400 treatments including antibiotics, oils, homeopathy, reiki, radionics, zero point energy, cleansing, diatomaceous earth, equimax, ivermetin, antiparisiticals, herbals, manuka honey and on and on and on. So many wonderful people have tried to help. I am so grateful to each and everyone. May God bless them all!

I went to a new primary care doctor, which my son recommended to me. She was young and a grad of the Yale Medical Program. Truthfully I didn't' expect much from her given the treatment most Morgies receive. At the first meeting, Dr. P was very pleasant. She asked me to undress, this was embarrassing for several reasons. One I was covered in sores and open wounds. Two I am very overweight now. Three there is no peer reviewed medical information to back this illness, and four the horror of my skin condition. She examined me, and at the end she looked me right in the eye and said, "No one should have to live like this." She cried and then said, "We have to fix this." Dr. P asked if she could photograph my hip, rear, and arm so that a dermatologist friend in Boston could give his opinion. I agreed. I went home with hope in my heart because of the compassion I had witnessed within this woman. I was joyful and cried myself. I didn't dread coming back for the follow up visit. Unfortunately, the second visit was completely different. Dr. P was very cold. She didn't look me in the eye. She addressed the thyroid and anemia issues but no mention of the elephant in the room. It felt like I didn't' exist. As she started to depart the exam room, I asked her if she sent the photos to the dermatologist. She replied yes. I asked what he thought, she answered "DOP." (Delusions of parasitosis) I thought to myself, the doctors are the ones who are delusional.

Later I had an oncologist from Missouri contact me and ask to see some of my photos. After viewing the pictures, he said he recognized many of the formations and was very enthusiastic, feeling he could help me to understand how to treat some of it. He worked at a cancer research hospital and asked if I would allow the research committee to review the pictures and to send samples for continued testing in the facility. I was thrilled. Yet after 2 months of no contact from the doctor, I received a message from someone else that he would no longer be able to help me and to discontinue any further contact. There is a theme here. There are other elements at play. Often at times Morgies will hear high pitched frequencies in their heads, as if a switch has been turned on. As easily as it is switched on, it also turns off in the same manner.

As the Morgellons moved more into my knees and hips I became unable to navigate the stairs. Walking with a cane became my "norm". I could go on and on about the pain, suffering, and isolation that come from this condition. Why are some of us so ill? Many people think we are all ill. Similar blood cells, fibers, and debris, are found in the chemtrails being sprayed. To quote others, "There is something about us that indicates, we are like the canaries in the gold mines. We react to it, whereas others don't." Perhaps we hailed from a different place. Perhaps we are sent here with a purpose of exposing and stopping this travesty. I know that some people, if they are people, know what it is and who made it. It did not evolve naturally over time.

A year ago when I heard about Christopher Macklin, I was in a terrible state. I had tried everything. My hip and rear area were deeply ingrained with a root system of vines, craters, and oozing flesh. It was difficult to sit, sleep, or walk. My arms were split open and had numerous sores. My shoulder had a large ravine area, a gaping hole which extended down the arm. My head was still shaved, for every time I tried to regrow my hair the polyurethane type material would start oozing, producing sores and the skin behind my ear would split open. I felt I would never see the end of this affliction. I often thought of Job in the Bible.

I was so excited when I first talked with Christopher. How blessed I was to be led to him. I began with sessions twice a week. I said the prayers of protection, incorporating these into my everyday life. At first I didn't feel the energy as he worked on me, but as time went along his healing could be felt as the changes in the body happened. He developed some new techniques for treating this condition. Other illnesses, like cancer and diabetes, he could eliminate rather quickly. Morgellons with its lime based co-infections, was a shrewd enemy designed to overcome whatever defense was mounted.

Christopher knew how to send in the angels! He tried new approaches, like switching the time and space continuum. Christopher developed a new process which he calls, tachyonization. He burns out the foreign debris in my body. The black material vacates my body and I am able to see the area that has been treated turn black. At that point the area will heal. He can then look inside the body and evaluate the progression of its healing. When these nano materials, bacteria, viruses, and fungus are leaving the cells, organs and bones, this system becomes full of toxic materials. Normally a person's body enters a hertz stage. This causes you to feel as if you have the flu. You run a temperature, become nauseous, your body aches, etc. The liver and kidneys become overwhelmed with these cast off toxins.

Christopher has the ability to clear away and cleanse out this garbage from our system, restoring its balance. When I feel dreadful, he is always there to help. He worked on me for 2 weeks straight, morning and night, to mount a strong front against this enemy. I believe about 20 other Morgies have now reached out for Christopher's help.

As for me, I have seen tremendous changes and improvements in my conditions, including with my asthma. Discomfort in the spine and joints has greatly improved. I no longer need my CPAP equipment to sleep at night. The restless legs have calmed. The quantity of fibers have greatly diminished. Six years of growths in my hip and rear have drawn in and are relinquishing the debris. Injuries this deep cannot be healed overnight, but it is NOW healing and pulling in. I haven't seen any live insects.

I am healing!!!!!!!!!!!

I am almost there. Christopher is an amazing healer. His joyful spirit, compassion, and unrelenting care are a true gift. I am so grateful for his sacrifice of time and energy. I am grateful that he has been there to get me through this last chapter.

To others:

There have been many people who have been angels to me on this earth. I am grateful for their love, compassion, and support. Many worked on me for years. There are friends and family all over the world who believe in and uplift me. My faith in my heavenly Father has never wavered.

If you feel you may have Morgellons and Lymes, don't give up!! You WILL prevail! We are not alone!

Count each and every blessing, over and over again. Fear can wash away our hope and joy. ***Refuse to let it!***

Let the pain and suffering enhance your love and compassion for others. *In this love, in this sharing, you will defeat "THEM," whomever they are.* Remember always, you are a part of God. He wants the best for you, as we do for our children!

Thank you God for sending Christopher to lead us to help!

Prayers

Always remember to say prayers with conviction. God likes a bit of feistiness.

Please check back to our website periodically, or sign-up for our newsletter in order to receive changes or additions to the following prayers.

HTTP://CHRISTOPHERMACKLINMINISTRIES.COM

Prayer of Protection

I am of God

I ground myself to the Earth

I command you, God,

to place a bubble of 5th dimensional,

Unconditional Love around me to protect me

from negative entities & any fractals thereof,

manipulations and any transmissional frequencies

that are not for my highest good,

through all space/time continuum in every dimension

I thank you, God,

and send you my Unconditional Love

So Be It
Amen

Pyramid Prayer of Protection

I am of God

I ground myself to the Earth

I command you, God, to create an Esoteric Pyramid
around me with me in the King's Chamber,
put on the Holy Grail and the Ark of the Covenant.

I program this pyramid with the blueprint of
my DNA and the Keys of Enoch,
so as not to allow anything except for my highest good
to enter

through all space/time continuum in any dimension

Dear God, I command that you align it now

and track the alignment with the changes

and the Earth's polarity and activate it now

I thank you, God,

and send you my Unconditional Love

So Be It
Amen

Prayer to Remove Radionic Manipulations from Computer & Electronic Equipment

I am of God

I ground myself to the Earth

I command you, God, to remove all the radionic manipulation from this computer that is not for my highest good

through all space/time continuum in every dimension

I bring all the people involved in this manipulation, no matter how remote, in every dimension

Before you, God,
for justice in only the way you know how.

I release them to you

with Unconditional Love & Forgiveness.

I thank you, God,

and send you my Unconditional Love

So Be It
Amen

Prayer to Block Out Luciferian Spirits & Frequencies from Multimedia

I am of God

I ground myself to the Earth

I command you God to remove all the luciferian spirits & vibrations from this multimedia

through all space/time continuum in every dimension

I bring all the people involved with the manipulation up through infinite levels and 20 billion light years away,

Before you, God,
for justice in only the way you know how.

I release them all to you, God,

with Unconditional Love and forgiveness

I thank you, God,

and send you my Unconditional Love

So be it
Amen

Recognition Prayer

I am of God

I ground myself to the earth

Dear God, I command that you show

this person in their true form

through all space/time continuum

in every dimension

I thank you, God,

and send you my Unconditional Love

So Be It
Amen

Prayer to Remove Spiritual Attack

I am of God

I ground myself to the earth

I command you, God, to remove all the negative remote viewers, remove all manipulations and transmissional frequencies that are not for my highest good

through all space/time continuum in every dimension

remove all the machines & redundancies creating these frequencies

up through infinite levels and up to 20 billion light years away

I bring all the people before you, God, for justice in only the way you know how.

I release them to you now with Unconditional Love and Forgiveness

I thank you, God, and send you my Unconditional Love

So Be It
Amen

Food Blessing

I am of God

I ground myself to the Earth

I command you, God, to correct & rebalance any

modifications made to this food that are not of God

optimize the nutritional value of this food,

remove all its toxins,

and bless the souls of the animals and plants that have

given their life to provide nutrition to my body

through all space/time continuum in every dimension

I thank you, God,

and send you my Unconditional Love

So Be It

Amen

The Merkabah Field Prayer of Protection

I am of God

I ground myself to the Earth

I command you God to create an esoteric merkaba field
around me

to protect me from any negative entities,
manipulations and transmissional frequencies that
are not for my highest good

Program this merkaba with the blueprint
of my DNA and the Keys of Enoch,
so as not to allow anything to enter except for my
highest good.

through all space/time continuum in every dimension

I thank you, God,

and send you my Unconditional Love

So Be It
Amen

Prayer to Neutralize & Remove Chemtrails

I am of God

I ground myself to the Earth

I command you, God, to neutralize and remove all the negative and harmful substances

contained in the Chemtrails above us

I command you to

alter the biological and molecular structure

to convert these trails into harmless water vapors

so as to protect all the humans, animals,

and plants that inhabit our 3rd Dimensional Universe

through all space/time continuum in every dimension

I thank you, God,

and send you my Unconditional Love

So Be It
Amen

Prayer to Release Any Cellular Memory or Esoteric Transference From Past Life

(say 3X or 9X for sacred numbers)

I am of God

I ground myself to the Earth

I come before you, God, for forgiveness

for anything I have done in any past life to Infinitum,

through all space & time in any dimension

that has been brought back into this lifetime

and is affecting me now.

I release it all to you now

I thank you, God,

and send you my Unconditional Love

So Be It
Amen

Prayer to Release Past Life Connection Issues

(say 3x or 9X for sacred numbers)

I am of God

I ground myself to the Earth

I come before you God for forgiveness

for anything I have done in any past life to infinitum

through all space/time continuum in every dimension

that has been brought back into this lifetime

and is affecting my relationship with (person's name).

I release it all to you now

I thank you, God,

and send you my Unconditional Love

So Be It
Amen

Prayer to Release Karma

I am of God

I ground myself to the earth

Dear God, I realize this person (name)

has wronged me and it is not for me to judge

him/her in any way,

Dear God, I bring this person before you

for justice in only the way you know how.

And I release him/her to you with

Unconditional Love and Forgiveness

through all space/time continuum

in every dimension

I thank you, God,

and send you my Unconditional Love

So Be It
Amen

Prayer to Remove Holographic Insert

I am of God

I ground myself to the Earth

I command you, God, to remove this holographic insert

from my current space/time continuum

in this dimension and

I bring all the people who created it

Before you God

for justice in only the way you know how.

I release them all to you now

with Unconditional Love and Forgiveness

I thank you, God,

and send you my Unconditional Love

So Be It
Amen

Emotional Release Prayer

I am of God

I ground myself to the earth

Dear God,

I bring (assailant's name) before you

for justice in only the way you know how.

I realize it's not for me to judge (assailant)

therefore I release (assailant) to you, God

with Unconditional Love and Forgiveness

through all space/time continuum

in every dimension

I thank you, God,

and send you my Unconditional Love

So Be It
Amen

Made in the USA
Charleston, SC
12 March 2016